THE WOMAN
I WANTED TO BE

ALSO BY DIANE VON FURSTENBERG

Diane: A Signature Life

Diane von Furstenberg's Book of Beauty

THE WOMAN
I WANTED TO BE

Diane von Furstenberg

SIMON &
SCHUSTER

London · New York · Sydney · Toronto · New Delhi

A CBS COMPANY

First published in Great Britain by Simon & Schuster UK Ltd, 2014
This paperback edition published by Simon & Schuster UK Ltd, 2015

A CBS COMPANY

5 7 9 10 8 6 4

Simon & Schuster UK Ltd
1st Floor
222 Gray's Inn Road
London WC1X 8HB

www.simonandschuster.co.uk

Simon & Schuster Australia, Sydney
Simon & Schuster India, New Delhi

A CIP catalogue record for this book
is available from the British Library

ISBN: 978-1-47114-029-7
eBook ISBN: 978-1-47114-030-3

Interior design by Ruth Lee-Mui
Jacket art (chain link print) © DVF Studio, LLC
Front cover photograph by Peter Lindbergh
Back flap photograph by Hans Dorsinville

Printed and bound by CPI Group (UK) Ltd, Croydon, CR0 4YY

To Alexandre, Tatiana, Talita, Antonia, Tassilo, and Leon.
I will always protect you.
And to Barry, for protecting all of us.

If you wish to be loved, love!

—*Seneca*

Contents

Acknowledgments

I want to thank all of the people who helped to bring this project to life.

Linda Bird Francke for her patience and dedication as she collected my memories and structured this book, and for her friendship for the last four decades.

Genevieve Ernst for reading and correcting it with me over and over and putting up with me and my endless changes.

I could not have done it without you both.

Alice Mayhew for her macro support and knowledge, and Andrew Wylie for being the best agent. Franca Dantes for her incredible archival skills, Peter Lindbergh for the cover photo, and Tara Romeo for her assistance with the cover design. Lisa Watson for transcribing my rambling, Jonathan Cox for keeping all of the chapters straight, and Liz McDaniel for helping with the book jacket.

THE WOMAN
I WANTED TO BE

Introduction

When I was a child, studying for my exams, I would pretend I was teaching imaginary students. It was my way to learn.

Living is learning, and as I look back at the many layers of experience I collected, I feel ready to share some of the lessons I learned along the way.

Living also means aging. The good thing about aging is that you have a past, a history. If you like your past and stand by it, then you know you have lived fully and learned from your life.

Those were the lessons that allowed me to be the woman I am.

As a girl, I did not know what I wanted to do but I knew the kind of woman I wanted to be. I wanted to be my own person, independent and free. I knew that freedom could only be achieved if I took full responsibility for myself and my actions, if I were true to truth, if I became my very best friend.

Life is not always a smooth ride. Landscapes change, people come in and out, obstacles appear and disrupt the planned itinerary, but one thing you know for sure is that you will always have yourself.

I have arranged this book into chapters on what has inspired me the most and continues to give me strength: family, love, beauty, and the business of fashion. But I must single out the person who was the most important in shaping my life, in making me the woman I wanted to be . . . my mother. That is where this memoir begins.

THE
WOMAN
I AM

1

ROOTS

There is a large frame on the bookshelf in my bedroom in New York. In it is a page torn from a German magazine of 1952. It is a photo of an elegant woman and her small daughter in the train station of Basel, Switzerland, waiting for the Orient Express. The little girl is nestled in her mother's tented coat and is eating a brioche. That was the first time, at the age of five, that I had my photo in a magazine. It is a sweet picture. My mother's older sister, Juliette, gave it to me when I was first married, but it is only recently that I realized its true importance.

On the surface, it is a photograph of a glamorous, apparently wealthy woman en route to a ski holiday with her curly-haired little girl. The woman is not looking into the camera, but there is a hint of a smile as she knows she is being photographed. Her appearance is elegant. Nothing would indicate that only a few years before, she was in another German-speaking railroad station coming back from the Nazi concentration camps where she had been a prisoner for thirteen months, a bunch of bones, close to death from starvation and exhaustion.

How did she feel when the photographer asked her name to be put in the magazine? Proud, I imagine, to be noticed for her style and elegance. Only seven years had passed. She was not a number anymore. She had a name; warm, beautiful, clean clothes; and most of all she had a daughter, a healthy little girl. "God has saved my life so that I can give you life," she used to write me every New Year on my birthday. "By giving you life, you gave me my life back. You are my torch, my flag of freedom."

My voice catches each time I speak publicly about my mother, and I do in every speech I make, aware that I wouldn't be giving that speech if Lily Nahmias had not been my mother. Sometimes it feels odd that I always bring up her story, but somehow I am compelled to. It explains the child I was, the woman I became.

"I want to tell you the story of a young girl who, at twenty-two years old, weighed fifty-nine pounds, barely the weight of her bones," I say to a seminar at Harvard about girls' health. "The reason she weighed fifty-nine pounds is that she had just spent thirteen months in the Nazi death camps of Auschwitz and Ravensbrück. It was a true miracle that that young girl didn't die, though she came very close. When she was liberated and returned to her family in Belgium, her mother fed her like a little bird, every fifteen minutes a tiny bit of food, and then a little bit more, making her feel as if she was being slowly blown up like a balloon. Within a few months her weight was close to normal."

There are always murmurs in the audience when I get to that point in my mother's story, perhaps because it is so shocking and unexpected or maybe because I am living history to a young audience that has heard only vaguely about Auschwitz. It must be hard to imagine the high-energy, healthy woman speaking to them having a mother who weighed fifty-nine pounds. Whatever it is, I want and need to honor my mother, her courage and her strength. It is what made me the woman she wanted me to be.

"God has saved my life so that I can give you life." Her words resonate with me every day of my life. I feel it is my duty to make up for all the suffering she endured, to always celebrate freedom and live fully. My birth was her triumph. She was not supposed to survive; I was not supposed to be born. We proved them wrong. We both won the day I was born.

I repeat a few of the lessons my mother drummed into me that have served me well. "Fear is not an option." "Don't dwell on the dark side of things, but look for the light and build around it. If one door closes, look for another one to open." "Never, ever, blame others for what befalls you, no matter how horrible it might be. Trust you, and only you, to be responsible for your own life." She lived those lessons. In spite of what she endured, she never wanted others to feel that she was a victim.

I didn't used to talk nearly as much about my mother. I took her for granted, as children do their mothers. It was not until she died in 2000 that I fully realized what an incredibly huge influence she had been on me and how much I owe her. Like any child, I hadn't paid much attention. "OK, OK, you told me that already," I'd brush her off, or even pretend not to hear. I bridled, too, at the unsolicited advice she persisted in giving my friends. In fact, it annoyed me. Now, of course, I feel I have had the experience and earned the wisdom to hand out my own unsolicited advice, and I press every lesson my mother taught me on my children, grandchildren, and anyone I talk to. I have become her.

I didn't know, as a very little girl in Brussels, why my mother had two lines of blue tattooed numbers on her left arm. I remember thinking they were some sort of decoration and wished I had them, too, so my arms wouldn't look so plain. I didn't understand why the housekeeper often told me not to bother her when she was lying down in her bedroom. I instinctively knew my mother needed her rest and I would tiptoe around the house so I wouldn't disturb her.

Sometimes I'd ignore the housekeeper's instructions and, gathering my beloved little picture books, I would sneak into her darkened room in the hope she would smile and read them to me. More often than not she did. She loved books and taught me to cherish them. She read my little picture books to me so many times I memorized them. One of my favorite things to do was to fake reading them, carefully turning the pages at the right time and showing off, pretending that I could read.

My mother was very strict. I never doubted that she loved me, but if I said something she didn't approve of or failed to live up to her expectations, she would give me a severe look or pinch me. I would be sent to the corner, my face to the wall. Sometimes I would go to the corner by myself, knowing I had done wrong. She spent a lot of time with me, sometimes playing, but mostly teaching me anything she could think of. She read me fairy tales and would tease me when I got scared. I remember how she amused herself by telling me that I was an abandoned child she had found in the garbage. I would cry until she took me in her arms, consoling me. She wanted me to be strong and not be afraid. She was very demanding. Before I had learned how to read, she had me memorize and recite the seventeenth-century fables of La Fontaine. As soon as I was old enough to write, she insisted I write stories and letters with perfect spelling and grammar. I remember how proud I was when she praised me.

To train me never to succumb to shyness, she made me give a speech at every family gathering, teaching me to be comfortable speaking in public no matter the audience. Like many children I was scared of the dark, but unlike most mothers, she shut me in a dark closet and waited outside so I would learn for myself that there was nothing to be afraid of. That was just one of the times she'd say "Fear is not an option."

My mother did not believe in coddling children too much or over-protecting them. She wanted me to be independent and responsible for myself. My earliest memories are of traveling with my parents and being left alone in the hotel room while they went out to dinner. I did not mind nor did I feel lonely. I was so proud that they trusted me to stay alone. I liked entertaining myself and feeling grown up. To this day, I have the same feeling and sense of freedom when I check into a hotel room alone.

When my parents allowed me to join them in a restaurant, my mother often encouraged me to get up and check out the room, and sometimes, even to go outside and report to her what I'd seen, who I had met. That instilled curiosity in me—watch what other people do, make friends with people I do not know. When I was nine, she sent me on the train from Brussels to Paris all by myself to visit her sister, my favorite aunt, Mathilde. I felt so proud to be responsible for myself. I think, deep down, I was a bit nervous, but I would never admit it and pride overcame the fear.

I still like to travel alone, and at times prefer it. Even on business trips, I don't like traveling with an entourage because it limits my freedom and reduces the fun of the unpredictable. I love the adventure, that feeling of excitement and satisfaction I had when I was a little girl. To be alone on the road, in an airport, with my bag, my passport, my credit cards, my phone, and a camera makes me feel so free and happy. I thank my mother for always encouraging me to "go."

Independence. Freedom. Self-reliance. Those were the values she was drumming into me, and she did it with such naturalness that I never questioned or resisted her. There was no other way but to be responsible for myself. As much as I loved and respected her, I was certainly a little frightened of her, and never wanted to displease her. I understand now that she was processing all of her past frustrations and unhappy experiences and putting them into a package of strength and positivity. That is the gift she prepared for me. It felt occasionally like a heavy burden, but I never questioned it, even if I sometimes wished I belonged to some other family.

Happily she let up on me somewhat when I was six and my baby brother, Philippe, was born. I adored him. To my surprise, having never played with dolls, I felt maternal, and to this day I think of him as my first child. As the older sister, I played with him and sometimes tortured him a bit, but as my mother had done to me, I taught him everything I knew and was very protective. When we played doctor, I asked him to urinate into a little bottle, only to then laugh at him that he had actually done it. We also used to play travel agency with my parents' airline brochures, scheduling and booking imaginary trips all over the world.

Philippe says he realized that I loved him the day I transcribed all the words from a Beatles record while I was at boarding school in England, and sent them to him. There were no computers then, no Internet, no iTunes, just a doting sister with pen and paper, listening to the lyrics and transcribing them. We're still extremely close, and he is still my baby brother, whom I always try to impress and tease. Philippe is a successful businessman in Brussels, has two amazing daughters, Sarah and Kelly, and his wife, Greta, launched and runs DVF Belgium. Philippe and I talk on the phone every weekend and whenever I miss my parents, I call him.

I don't think my mother was half as hard on him as she'd been with me. He was a boy, after all, and we are much softer and less demanding toward boys in our family. It was I she related to, the daughter she was determined would survive whatever life threw at her. As I grew older, I understood. Independence and freedom were key to her because she had lost both. Self-reliance had kept her alive.

My mother was twenty and engaged to my father in 1944 when the Nazi SS arrested her on May 17 for working in the Belgian Resistance. She was living in a "safe house" and her job was to go around Brussels on her bicycle to deliver documents and fake papers to those who needed them. Immediately after her arrest, she was thrown onto a crowded truck, which took her and many other suspected saboteurs to a prison in Malines, Flanders, a city twenty-five kilometers from Brussels. To avoid being tortured into giving information about others in the resistance, she said she knew nothing and that she was hiding in the safe house because she was Jewish. The woman who was interrogating her advised her not to say she was Jewish. She ignored it and was deported on the twenty-fifth transport, which left Malines on May 19, 1944. She was sent to Auschwitz and given prisoner number 5199.

My mother often told me how she'd written her parents a note on a scrap of paper and dropped it from the truck onto the street. She hoped but had no idea whether anyone ever picked it up and delivered it. It wasn't until after her death that I found out that the message had been delivered. I'd loaned the house she'd owned on Harbour Island in the Bahamas to my first cousin Salvator. Salvator left me a thick envelope full of family photographs, in the midst of which was a sealed envelope marked "Lily, 1944." Inside was a piece of torn paper with faint handwriting. I stared at it until I finally made out the words:

> *Dear Mommy and Daddy,*
>
> *I am writing to tell you that your little Lily is leaving. Where, she does not know, but God is everywhere isn't he? So she will never be alone or unhappy.*
>
> *I want you both to be courageous, and not forget that you have to be in good health for my wedding. I am counting more than ever in having a beautiful ceremony.*
>
> *I want you to know that I am leaving with a smile, I promise. I love you very very much and will soon kiss you more than ever.*
>
> Your little daughter,
Lily

I couldn't breathe. Could I be holding the actual note my mother had told me she had written to her parents on that truck, using a burnt match for a pencil? On the other side of the note was a plea for anybody finding the piece of paper to please deliver it to her parents' address. Somebody had found it and delivered it to her parents and my aunt Juliette, Salvator's mother, had kept it in a sealed envelope all these years!

I was in shock; I'd only half-believed her story of the note. All these stories about her arrest and deportation seemed surreal, more like a movie script, and yet they were true. She had always told me that she was more worried about her parents than herself. I held the proof in my shaky hands.

I walked out of the house in a daze and across the beach into the clear blue water. "This explains who I am," I said out loud to myself. "I am the daughter of a woman who went to the concentration camps with a smile."

The sayings she had drummed into me as a child and which had sometimes annoyed me took on whole new meanings. She had often illustrated one of her favorites—"you never really know what is good for you; what may seem the absolute worst thing to happen to you can, in fact, be the best"—by her story of the inhuman train ride to Auschwitz and her arrival.

No food. No water. No air. No toilet. Four days jammed in a cattle car. An "older woman" in her forties who spoke a little German comforted my mother and gave her a sense of protection. My mother made sure never to leave her side, especially when they arrived at Auschwitz and were unloaded onto a ramp. Women with children were immediately separated from the rest and sent toward long, low buildings while the others were forced into a long line. At the head of the line, a soldier directed the prisoners into two groups. Looking on, from the top of the ramp, was an officer in white.

When it came her turn, the older woman was directed to the group being formed on the left and my mother quickly followed her. The soldier did not stop her, but the white-coated officer, who had not interfered until then, did. Striding down the ramp, he walked directly to my mother, yanked her away from her friend, and threw her into the group on the right. My mother always said that she'd never felt such sheer hatred for anyone as she felt for that man.

That man was Dr. Josef Mengele, she found out later, the notorious Angel of Death, who killed or mutilated many, many prisoners in medical experiments, especially children and twins. Why did he go through the trouble of saving her? Did she remind him of someone he cared about? However evil or not his intentions were, he saved her life. The group the older woman was assigned to went directly to the gas chamber. The group my mother was thrust into did not.

I always use that story when I want to console anyone, just as my mother told it so often to me: You never know how something that seems the worst thing turns out to be the best.

After that, she was determined to survive, no matter the horror. Even when the unmistakable smell of the smoke coming from the camp crematorium seemed unbearable and her fellow prisoners would say "We're all going to die," my mother would insist: "No, we're not. We're going to live." Fear was not an option.

Nearly one million Jews were murdered at Auschwitz, many in the gas chamber. Others were executed, or killed in Dr. Mengele's experiments, or died from starvation and exhaustion from slave labor. My mother was fortunate, if anyone could have been considered fortunate in those unimaginably cruel surroundings. She was put to work on the twelve-hour night shift in the nearby weapons factory making bullets; so long as she worked she was useful and was kept alive. She was tiny, barely five feet tall, and naturally slender. She had never eaten much and could exist, albeit barely, on the miniscule rations of bread and watery soup she and other prisoners were given. Heavier prisoners, radically deprived of anything close to the amount of food they were used to, she told me, were the first to succumb to starvation.

If ever I think I'm too lazy to do a necessary chore, if I hesitate to go out because of the cold or complain about having to wait in line, I remember my mother. I envision her being marched out of Auschwitz with sixty thousand others in the winter of 1945, just nine days before the Soviet troops reached the camp. The SS hastily executed thousands of inmates and marched the others fifty kilometers through the snow to a train depot where they were stuffed into freight cars and sent to Ravensbrück in the north, and from there force-marched again to their new camps, in my mother's case to Neustadt-Glewe in Germany. Some fifteen thousand prisoners died on that Death March, of exposure, exhaustion, illness, or being shot by the SS for falling or lagging behind.

In what can only be described as a miracle, my tiny mother survived it all. She was one of the 1,244 who survived the camps out of the 25,631 Belgian Jews who were deported. Her will and spirit to live were her defiance of the evil she had endured, a declaration of her future. When Neustadt-Glewe was liberated a few months later by the Russians, followed closely by the Americans, my mother's weight was barely the weight of her bones.

She was hospitalized at an American base and wasn't expected to live. She defied the odds again. When she was stable enough to return home to Belgium she had to fill out a form, as did all survivors returning to their countries. I found that form. It had her name and date of birth on it and a question: "in what condition" she was returning from her thirteen months in captivity. Her astonishing answer was, in impeccable handwriting: "en très bonne santé" ("in very good health").

My father, Leon Halfin, was very different from my mother. Where she was strict and somewhat distant, he was relaxed and affectionate. In his eyes I could do no wrong and he loved me unconditionally. As a child I loved him much more than my demanding mother, though maybe I respected her a little more. When I needed to get up to go to the bathroom in the middle of the night, I would call for my father and that made him laugh. "Why do you call me and not your mother?" he'd ask. And I would reply: "Because I don't want to disturb her."

My father never scolded me. He simply adored me and I adored him. I was as affectionate toward him as he was to me. I loved to sit on his lap, covering him with kisses and drinking all of his after-dinner lemon tea. To my father I was the most beautiful thing in the world and I felt entitled to his love and devotion.

My father and I looked alike and we had the same kind of relentless energy. He loved American cars, and when I was nine or ten he would often take me for a drive in his beautiful, sky-blue and navy American Chevrolet Impala convertible, a bicolor combination that was very popular in the late fifties. In that era, before seat belts were common, I would kneel on the front seat instead of sitting, because I thought that that would make people think I was a grown-up. I always, always wanted to be older than my age. I never wanted to be a little girl. I wanted to be a woman, a sophisticated woman, a glamorous woman. I wanted to be important.

My father, unknowingly, hastened that wish. When he came to say good night to me and kiss me in my bed, he was often cautioned by my mother. "Be careful, don't wake up her senses," she'd say. My father used to think my mother's warning was hysterically funny. How could he, a man, wake up the senses of a little girl? Looking back now, however, no matter how funny he thought it was, he did wake up my senses. My father made me feel like a woman, so my mother was clever actually to say that.

The feelings were not sexual. It was the awareness that he was a man and that my relationship with him was therefore different from one I'd have with a woman. How lucky I was that this first man in my life loved me uncritically, unguardedly, without judging. I did not have to work for his love, I did not have to please him; his approval required no effort. That made an important impact on my life, and though I didn't know it then, I now know it has made my relationships with men much easier. What I owe my father, and what I am so thankful for, is how comfortable I always feel with men. He gave me confidence.

That first love and affection marks the way I presume men feel toward me. I simply take their fondness for granted, neither expecting nor looking for it. The biggest gift my father gave me was not to be needy. I had so much love from him that I didn't really need any more. In fact, I sometimes had to push it away because his display of affection in front of people embarrassed me.

My father was a successful businessman, a distributor of General Electric electronic tubes and semiconductors. He did well, so we lived very comfortably.

My parents were a striking couple. My father was very good-looking with high cheekbones and a mischievous smile. My mother had an elegant build and beautiful legs. She dressed very well and had a lot of allure. She was very much the boss of the house and I always saw her as the brains of the family. As much as I adored my father it was to her I went for advice.

She was not a traditional housewife, and only on Sundays, the housekeeper's day off, did I occasionally see her in the kitchen. She would make a delicious grilled chicken with crispy potatoes and my father would bring pastries for dessert. My favorite petit gâteau was called a Merveilleux and was made of meringue, chocolate, and whipped cream. We were, after all, in Belgium, the land of chocolate. In fact, most of what my mother did at home was to instruct everyone else, but she did it very well. Our apartment was beautifully decorated, full of antiques she had collected. I have a clear memory of her looking for and finally finding the Empire chandelier she so desired. It now illuminates my Mayfair shop in London.

Since my mother died, my father having died six years before, I have searched for clues in my parents' lives as to what formed them and why I am who I am. That quest has taken me to Eastern Europe and the city of Kishinev, then the capital of Bessarabia, now the capital of Moldova, where my father was born in 1912, and to Salonika, Greece, where my mother was born in 1922.

Both my parents' families were in the textile business. My father's father, a wealthy Russian merchant whose relatives included many intellectuals and artists—one relative, Lewis Milestone, directed the 1930 Academy Award–winning war film *All Quiet on the Western Front*—owned several fabric stores in Kishinev. My mother's father, Moshe Nahmias, a Sephardic Jew (a Jew of Spanish origin), moved his family from Salonika to Brussels when my mother was seven and ran La Maison Dorée, the large department store owned by his brother-in-law, Simon Haim. My maternal grandmother's sister, my great-aunt Line, was married to the wealthy Simon Haim and had urged her sister to join her in Brussels with her family. So, although I had never made the connection before, I do indeed have a legacy of the fashion and retail business from both sides of my family.

There is nothing I could find in my mother's childhood that would give her the unimaginable strength to survive the death camps. As far as I could tell, she had a pleasant, uneventful young life in Brussels, rather spoiled as the youngest of three girls in the family. The only challenge for her and her two older sisters, who had gone to an Italian school in Greece, was to become more fluent in French when they moved to Brussels so they could do well at school. My maternal grandparents, who spoke Ladino, the language of the Sephardic Jews, at home, changed the birthdates of the girls when the family arrived in Brussels, passing them off as two years younger so they would have more time to adapt, learn French, and be successful at school. My mother went to the Lycée Dachsbeck, the same school I went to years later, and we even had the same kindergarten teacher and the same headmistress, Mademoiselle Gilette. I found out recently that Mlle. Gilette had ignored the racial laws of the Nazi occupation and allowed my mother to graduate from high school. It is probably why she chose me to blow out the candles on the cake at the school's seventy-fifth anniversary in 1952; I was the daughter of an alumna who went to the death camps and survived.

My father arrived in Brussels two years after my mother and her family moved to Belgium. He was seventeen in 1929 and was planning to follow in his brother's footsteps and train to be a textile engineer, when something went very wrong in Kishinev. My grandfather's business went bankrupt, which actually killed him, and my grandmother was no longer able to send money to my future father. He stopped studying, although I am not sure he ever officially entered school in Belgium, and went to work, taking any job he could find. He had no plan to go back home and enjoyed his freedom as a young, good-looking man even though his life as a refugee was not always easy.

It was the war that brought my parents together. When Germany invaded and occupied Belgium in 1940, many people fled south in what was called L'Exode. Thousands of cars jammed the roads escaping from the occupation. My father and his best friend, Fima, drove south to France and settled, temporarily, in a small hotel in Toulouse. They were young and very handsome and even though it was wartime and the situation was serious, they laughed a lot and had many women along the way. My mother also arrived in Toulouse with her aunt Line and uncle Simon. They made the trip rather regally in a Cadillac with a driver.

Fima had money but my father did not. He hated being dependent on his friend, so every morning he went around on a bicycle looking for the jobs that had been posted, but in every place he arrived, the job had been taken. "Try the train station," a sympathetic would-have-been employer suggested. There he met a man named Jean who began the sequence of events that would draw my mother and father together.

"I know someone who needs to go back to Belgium and has to sell a very large amount of dollars because Belgium won't allow anyone to bring in foreign currency," Jean told him. "Do you know anyone who wants to buy dollars? He paid thirty-four French francs for them and is willing to sell at thirty-three." My father certainly didn't know anyone who wanted to buy dollars, so he paid little attention. A few days later, completely by accident, he met another man called Maurice who had a friend looking to buy dollars and was willing to pay a rate of seventy-six French francs for them.

My father couldn't believe his ears. Was he understanding right? Jean had a seller at thirty-three and Maurice had a buyer at seventy-six. So much profit could be made with the difference. The problem was that my father had no idea how to find Jean. He didn't know his last name or where he lived, so he raced around Toulouse on his bicycle for three days and three nights, looking for him. On the fourth day, my father went to the cinema and, realizing he had left his newspaper when he came out of the theater, went back for it—and bumped into Jean!

It took days to smooth out the many complications and finalize the transaction, because the sum was very large and my father had to prove he could deliver the money. He had to borrow some from his friend Fima to do a small sample transaction first, to prove he was trustworthy and, after a few days, completed the whole exchange. Overnight he went from having no money at all to actually being rich. In his diary my father recalls feeling so ashamed of his worn-out suit during the transaction that the day it was completed he bought three suits, six shirts, and two pairs of shoes. His good fortune didn't end there. As fate would have it, the man who was buying the dollars turned out to be my mother's uncle Simon. And that is how my parents met.

Theirs was not an immediate romance. Leon Halfin was twenty-nine, ten years older than my mother, and very interested in being a ladies' man. But Lily was a Jewish girl, and as far as he was concerned, you didn't touch Jewish girls—you married them.

The news from Belgium was that things weren't so bad under the German occupation, and in October 1941, my parents returned separately to Belgium. My mother couldn't go to university because of the racial laws, so she went to fashion school, studied millinery, and learned how to make hats. My father, who now had a lot of money, did not go back to Tungsram, the electronics company he had worked for, but became an independent businessman in the radio field in Brussels. They saw each other at gatherings of older relatives and family friends, but my father always treated my mother like a little girl, teasing her and pinching her cheeks. There was no romance although they clearly liked each other. Leon didn't know my mother had a secret crush on him.

It wasn't until the summer of 1942, when the SS started rounding up Jews in Belgium and deporting them that the danger began in earnest. Lucie, my father's very good friend and ex-colleague at Tungsram, advised him to get out of Belgium and flee to Switzerland.

He bought fake papers from the Belgian underground and began to plan his escape under the assumed and typical Belgian name of Leon Desmedt. He did not go alone. Lucie arranged for Gaston Buyne, a nineteen-year-old Christian boy to accompany him through France to the Swiss border. In a surprising turn of events, they were joined by Renée, a nineteen-year-old girl my father had just met. She was a Belgian Catholic girl who had fallen in love with my father and wanted to run away with him. Her mother had recently died and she didn't like the woman her father had taken up with. That was the unlikely trio who set out together on August 6, 1942.

The train ride to Nancy, where they would transfer to another train to Belfort, was very dangerous. Gaston, a Belgian with legal papers, carried a lot of Leon's money—banknotes in his shoulder pads, gold coins in his shoes and socks, and more Swiss notes in his toiletry bag. Because Gaston looked Jewish, much more so than Leon, he turned out to be the perfect foil. There were many, many checkpoints at which the German SS would randomly order male passengers to pull down their trousers to check whether they were circumcised. Gaston was ordered to drop his pants. "Sorry," the SS man apologized to him, and didn't bother with my father who was sitting next to him.

They arrived in Nancy at night and checked into a hotel. The train to Belfort left at 5:15 a.m. and they had another run-in on board with a young SS soldier who wanted both Gaston and Leon to drop their pants. This time it was Renée who saved Leon by smiling coquettishly at the young soldier until he moved on to other passengers.

Belfort was even more dangerous. There were many, many Jewish refugees checking into the same hotel, but my father's fake ID saved him. The German SS raided the hotel that night and arrested all the Jews, but not Leon Desmedt. (My father's diary records that he made love to Renée twice that night.) Later they heard that all the people arrested that night were killed.

Leon and Renée parted ways with Gaston the next morning as they approached the Swiss border. They took a bus to Hérimoncourt, at which point Leon hired a local guide to lead them through the mountains and pastures into Switzerland just six kilometers away. That last leg of the escape cost fifteen hundred French francs with no guarantee of success. A few more refugees joined in as they met the guide at five a.m., among them a woman with a baby. She gave the baby a sleeping pill so he wouldn't cry, and they set out on foot through the alpine mountains to the border. "Run, run, run in that direction," the guide pointed and sent them off on their own. I remember my father telling me that it was the cows and their noisy bells that made their escape possible. By following the bells, Leon and Renée arrived at the Swiss border town of Damvant on August 8, 1942.

"Why do you carry so much money?" the border police asked my father. He told them that he was an industrialist from Belgium, but the police did not believe his story. "Your papers are fake," they said. They confiscated his money but did allow him to enter Switzerland. "You can claim it back when you leave," the police told him.

My father was very lucky. Although he remained under surveillance by the Swiss authorities, and was unable to travel freely or have access to his money without going through long bureaucratic requests, he spent a few fairly pleasant years there. He separated from Renée, who eloped with a policeman soon after their arrival, and began to miss Lily, the vivacious "little" girl he'd left behind in Belgium. The occupation of Brussels had become very severe and he was worried about her. Lily and her parents had to abandon their apartment and live separately. She was hiding in a resistance house where she worked. My aunt Juliette sent her son, my cousin Salvator, to live with his Christian Belgian nanny.

Curious Lily went to her family's apartment one day and discovered that the SS had ransacked it and stolen all their belongings. She also discovered something that would change her life. There was a letter in the mailbox, an unexpected letter from Switzerland, from Leon, the man she had met in Toulouse and never forgotten. After reading and rereading it many times, she responded. It started a daily correspondence between them, carefully crafted because all the letters had to go through censors as the wide blue stripe across the stationery indicated. I am lucky to possess those letters, which, over time, became more and more intimate and passionate. They wrote about their love and about the moment they would meet again after the war, that they would marry, build a life together, have a family, and be happy forever. It was all about hope and love.

Then, suddenly, Lily's letters stopped. (It was then, I recall my father telling me, that the mirror in his bedroom, on which he had taped a photo of my mother, fell and broke.)

He wrote to her again and again, begging in vain for an answer. On July 15, two months after my mother's arrest, he received a letter from Juliette, my mother's older sister, written in code to get through the censors.

"Dear Leon," she wrote. "I have very bad news. Lily has been hospitalized."

When my mother returned from Germany in June 1945, my father was still in Switzerland. By the time he came back to Brussels four months later, she had gained back much of the weight she had lost, but she wasn't the same naïve, mischievous, fun-loving, passionate girl he had been corresponding with and planned to marry. That girl was gone forever. This new young woman had endured true horrors and would carry the wounds forever.

In his diary, my father wrote with great honesty about their re-union. He admitted that he barely recognized the girl he had been separated from for more than two years. She was different, a stranger to him. Lily sensed his unease and told him he was under no obliga-tion to marry her. The love was still there, he reassured her as he hid his doubts away. They were married on November 29, 1945.

The doctor warned them, "No matter what, you have to wait a few years before having a baby. Lily isn't strong enough for childbirth and the baby may not be healthy." Six months later, I was accidentally conceived. Remembering the doctor's warning, both my mother and father were concerned. They thought they could get rid of the preg-nancy by taking long rides on his motorcycle over the cobblestoned streets, but it didn't work. Finally one morning my father brought home some pills to induce a miscarriage. My mother threw those pills out the window.

I was born healthy and strong in Brussels on New Year's Eve, December 31, 1946, a miracle. Because of the price my mother paid for that miracle, I never felt I had the right to question her, complain, or make her life more difficult. I was always a very, very good little grown-up girl, and for some reason felt it was my role to protect her. In his diaries, my father confesses that at first he was disappointed that I was not a boy, but within a few days he had totally accepted me and fallen in love with my mother again.

I have long suspected that if I hadn't been born, my mother might have killed herself. If nothing else, my existence gave her a focus and a reason to keep going. For all the strength and determination of her personality, she was extremely fragile. She hid it very well, and when people were around she was always light and fun. But when she was alone, she was often overtaken by uncontrollable sadness. When I came home from school in the afternoons, I would sometimes find her sitting in her darkened bedroom, weeping. Other times, when she picked me up from school, she'd take me to have a patisserie, or antiques shopping, laughing with me and giving no hint of her painful memories.

The people who went to the camps didn't want to talk about it and the people who weren't in the camps didn't want to hear about it, so I sensed she often felt like a stranger or an alien. When she did talk about it to me, she would only emphasize the good—the friendships, the laughter, the will to go back home and the dream of a plate of spaghetti. If I asked her how she endured, she would joke and say, "Imagine it is raining and you run in between the drops!" She always told me to trust the goodness of people. She wanted to protect me, but I realized that it is also how she protected herself . . . denying the bad . . . always denying the bad and demanding that the good forces win and, no matter what, never appearing a victim.

She did the best she could to put the war behind her. She had the two sets of tattooed numbers removed. And in a wonderful gesture of defiance, and to override her memory of the bitter cold she'd endured, she bought a very expensive, warm sable coat with the restitution money she got from the German government.

I spent a lot of time alone as a child, reading and imagining a grand life for myself. My childhood went smoothly, though life in Brussels was often gray and boring. I loved my big school, I loved my books, and I was a very good student. I loved my brother and my girlfriends,

Mireille Dutry and Myriam Wittamer, whose parents owned the best patisserie in Brussels. On the weekends, our family spent Sundays in the country at my great-great-aunt and -uncle's villa. They had a beautiful house on the edge of a large forest, the Forêt de Soignes. I loved walking in the woods, picking chestnuts in the winters and berries in the summers. My father would play cards with the men and my mother gossiped with the women. We ate a lot of good food. On the long, gray days, I lost myself reading Stendhal, Maupassant, Zola, and, on a lighter note, my favorite, *The Adventures of Tintin,* comic books about a daring young boy reporter created by the Belgian cartoonist Hergé. I lived vicariously through Tintin's travels and exploits. Would I ever discover all these exotic places in the world? It seemed like nothing would ever happen to me.

When I had a few days off from school and my parents could not travel, I would often visit my aunt Mathilde in Paris. She had an elegant boutique off the Faubourg Saint-Honoré catering to a loyal, international clientele. She sold printed cashmere sweaters and jersey dresses and suits. I would spend entire days in the shop. My job was to fold the clothes and put them back in order. It was my first encounter with fashion, retail, and the secret virtues of jersey fabrics.

In Paris, I also visited my cousins, Eliane and Nadia Neiman, the two daughters of my father's rich cousin Abraham, who had invented the theft alarm for cars. The girls spoke perfect Russian, gave piano recitals, and were very sophisticated. I felt terribly awkward and provincial when I visited them for tea or lunch at their villa in Neuilly. During the summers, my brother and I would go to summer camp near Montreux in the Swiss Alps or in the North Sea resort of Le Coq-sur-Mer in Belgium. We would also go on trips with my parents and my aunts and uncles to the South of France or the Swiss mountains.

My parents were a good-looking couple, and they loved each other very much, but my father wasn't as sensitive around my mother as he should have been. He didn't want to acknowledge her wounds, so he ignored them. He was a hardworking, generous man, but he could be indifferent and sometimes verbally harsh. I don't think he had any real love affairs after he married my mother. He traveled frequently on business, and I am sure he did not always spend his nights alone, but that was not the problem between my parents. It was his insensitivity toward her that made her feel vulnerable. So the scene was set for what came next. And what came next was a man named Hans Muller.

The letter, addressed to my mother, was on the table in our front hall that day when I came back from school. For reasons that I still cannot fathom, I opened the blue envelope with the very clear handwriting. It was from someone named Hans Muller, who, I realized as I read, was a friend of hers. I did not know who this Hans was and I do not recall what the letter said, but I remember that my heart started to beat fast. I felt something major had happened, something that would change all of our lives, and that something was Hans. Knowing I had done something wrong, I carefully put the letter back in the blue envelope and left it on the table, but the damage was done. My mother came home, saw the envelope, and I confessed I'd opened it. I had never seen her so upset and angry. Though I was twelve at the time, she reacted in a very violent way, slapping me across the face with all her strength. I was desperate, I was in pain, I was ashamed. Whatever had come upon me to open that letter?

My face was only a little bruised the next day when I went to class, but my insides were crushed. I had disappointed my mother. I had betrayed her trust. We never discussed it again and I am not sure what she told my father that night when he came home. Was he home anyway or was he traveling? I don't remember. I felt terrible, and to this day I have never again opened a letter or looked at a document or an email that was not addressed to me.

The following year, over my father's objections but to my own excitement, my mother sent me to Pensionnat Cuche, a private boarding school by the Lake Sauvabelin in Lausanne, Switzerland. It did not escape me that Lausanne is very close to Geneva, where Mr. Muller lived.

During the two wonderful years I spent at that school, living my own life, making many friends, and for the first time relishing my independence from my parents, I pieced together the story of my mother and Hans Muller. My father traveled a lot for his business, often taking my mother with him. When the travel entailed planes, they flew separately as insurance for my brother and me in case anything happened.

Hans Muller was my mother's seatmate on one of those trips, a long flight from Brussels to New York. He was a very handsome young Swiss German businessman who worked in the fruit business. Separated from his wife, he lived with his small son, Martin, who was the same age as my brother, Philippe. Monsieur Muller was polite and considerate, a stark contrast to my father, whose manners could be coarse and who sometimes belittled my mother in public. Hans was quite a bit younger than my mother and very taken with her. He would tell me, over the years, that he had never met a woman so attractive, interesting, and intelligent. They developed a friendship, which eventually led to a secret love affair and later to a long relationship.

I was not happy when my father insisted I be brought back to Brussels after my two years at boarding school in Switzerland. There I was, stuck at home again, and not a pleasant home at all. My mother and my father argued all the time and there was a lot of tension. I was relieved when they decided to officially separate. I think they both expected me to be upset that the family was splitting up. I wasn't, but I felt sad for my little brother. He was only nine and my parents would continue to fight over him for years after their separation and divorce.

As for me, I was fifteen in 1962. I felt grown up and secure, eager for whatever change lay ahead. Never once did I make my mother feel guilty about leaving my father, but instead I encouraged her and supported her completely. What she wanted, I'm convinced, was her freedom and independence after sixteen years of marriage, and I felt she deserved it. Was Hans an excuse or the reason? I never knew for sure. "Go on," I said. In turn, she would never make me feel guilty about anything either. When, years later, I told her I was leaving my husband, Egon, her response was "All right" and that was the end of it.

My father was devastated when my mother left him. His whole life revolved around his work and his family. I was not very sympathetic. Though I looked exactly like him and I loved him so very much, it was my mother I identified with. She wanted to move on, to experience life, to travel, learn, grow, expand her horizons, meet people, live her life. I understood it.

And so my parents parted and my childhood ended. One door closed, many others opened. I went on to another boarding school, this one in England, for two years and later to the University of Madrid in Spain. My mother lived with Hans for the next twenty years before separating from him, too. And I, with my mother as my role model, started to become the woman I wanted to be.

If anyone had the right to be bitter, my mother did, but never, ever did I hear her express any bitterness. She looked for the good in everything and everyone.

I'm often asked what was the worst thing that ever happened to me, what were my biggest challenges. I find it difficult to answer because I have this habit I inherited from my mother that somehow transforms what's bad into something good, so in the end, I don't remember what was bad. When I have an obstacle in front of me, especially of someone else's making, I say "OK. I don't like it, but I can't change it, so let's find a way around it." Then I find a different path to a solution, which so satisfies me that I forget what the problem was in the first place. Of all the lessons my mother drummed into me, that was perhaps the most important. How could you possibly better yourself if you didn't face your challenges up front or if you laid your problems off on someone or something else and didn't learn from them? I offer that lesson often in my talks to young women. "Don't blame your parents, don't blame your boyfriend, don't blame the weather. Accept the reality, embrace the challenge, and deal with it. Be in charge of your own life. Turn negatives into positives and be proud to be a woman."

It doesn't happen overnight, of course, and I never stopped learning from my mother. Over and over, she reinforced the lessons she'd taught me as a child.

When I was in my thirties, I suddenly developed a fear of flying, but when I told her I was afraid, she looked at me, smiling, and said, "Tell me, what does it mean to be afraid?" When once I was conflicted about starting a new business, she said, "Don't be ridiculous. You know how to do it." When I was diagnosed with cancer at forty-seven, predictably she told me not to worry, that I had nothing to fear. I wanted to believe her, but I had my doubts. Because she never showed any sign even in private that she was afraid, I wasn't either. When my treatment was all done, she collapsed, and I realized that she had, in fact, been afraid for me, but by never showing it to me, she had made me strong and trusting that I would be fine.

After Egon and I married in 1969, she spent several months each year living with us in New York and formed close, loving relationships with my children, Alexandre and Tatiana. Her relationship with them was very different from the relationship she had had with me. She had never been very affectionate to me and there had always been a distance between us. As a result, I was reserved around her and never told her my intimate thoughts, except in letters. It was much easier for me to open up in letters, and I think easier for her, too. In her letters to me at boarding school in Switzerland and then in England, she would often call me her "pride," but actually she never told me that to my face until much, much later when she was about to die.

She was much more open with my daughter as a grandmother and my daughter was more open with her than with me. They had an amazing complicity and spent hours together on her bed, telling each other stories. Tatiana became an excellent storyteller and filmmaker.

My mother was superb at handling money. She had taken half my father's assets with her when she left him and invested them so well that she was, in her later years, able to feel secure and buy herself a beautiful house on the beach in Harbour Island, Bahamas. Had she been born at a different time and under different circumstances, she would have made a sought-after investment banker.

My son, Alexandre, benefited greatly from her financial skills. She taught him what stocks and bonds were, what kinds of companies were good investments, and about yields and dividends. Every afternoon when he came home from school, the two of them studied the stock market pages in the afternoon edition of the *New York Post* so he could see which stocks were going up and which down. When he was six or seven, my new boyfriend, Barry Diller, wanted to give him one share of stock for his birthday and told him he could choose which one. "Choose the most expensive," my mother advised him. Alexandre chose IBM.

There is no doubt the financial education she gave him turned him into the financier he is today. He manages the family money, sits on prestigious boards, and has proven to be a superb adviser to all of us.

My mother was my rock. For all that I thought I'd conquered my fear of flying, I remember a very scary, bumpy flight to Harbour Island with her and Alexandre when she had just gotten out of the hospital. When the plane dropped suddenly and made loud creaking noises, I closed my eyes and thought, "OK, I am afraid. Where do I go for strength? Do I take the hand of my big, strong son or of my weak, dying mother?" And there was no question that I would go to my mother for strength. I put my hand over hers.

At about the same time as that plane trip, I remember being anxious when my daughter, Tatiana, was about to give birth. It's one thing when your son has a child, but for some reason, when your daughter has a child, you feel it in your own flesh. It is physical agony. I was frightened for my little girl, thinking of all the things that could go wrong. I called my mother, in tears, while driving to the hospital. She was very frail, but she summoned the strength to make me strong, though happily it turned out I didn't need it. Antonia was born without any complication and Tatiana was fine. In yet another testament to her strength, my mother clung to life so that she could see Tatiana's baby. Though her body was almost nonexistent, her mind and her will were strong. So many times in her life she was ill and on the verge of dying, but her incredible strength and determination kept her alive.

We had already welcomed her first great-grandchild, Talita, the daughter of Alexandre and his then wife, Alexandra Miller, and just as intense in my memory is the astonishing day when Alexandre brought the one-year-old Talita in her carriage to visit me and my mother in the Carlyle hotel in New York. It was Mother's Day and Alexandre gallantly brought each of us a bouquet of flowers. All our eyes were on the adorable little girl who pulled herself upright, clinging to a chair, then suddenly launched off on her own and took her first steps! We all clapped and praised her, but then something unbelievable took place. I was watching my old mother, wrinkled and sick in her chair, looking at this little girl on the floor and that little girl looking back at her, when suddenly I saw a flash of something white, almost like lightning coming out of my mother and going into Talita. I believe that that day my mother's energy and spirit transferred to my granddaughter. I saw it happen, that white flash going from my mother into Talita. I saw it.

My mother did not die peacefully. I think she was reliving the horrors of the camps and fighting giving in to death, as she had in Auschwitz. It was not the first time she'd relived those horrors. As much as she had tried to bury the past and concentrate on looking forward to life, she had had a breakdown twenty years before during a visit to Germany with Hans and some clients of his. My heart had nearly stopped when Hans called me in New York to tell me he'd woken up that morning in the hotel to find my mother missing. He'd finally found her hiding in the lobby of the hotel, underneath the concierge's desk, disoriented, speaking loudly and making little sense. "Why? What happened?" I'd asked him, in a panic myself. He thought it must have been the dinner they'd had the night before with his clients at a restaurant. It was very hot and the people at the tables around her were speaking loudly in German. I suspected that she and Hans had also had a fight, but whatever the reason, she'd completely come apart.

Hans thought she might snap out of it if I talked to her and I tried to talk calmly to her over the phone, but all she could do was babble nonsensically. Hans drove her back to Switzerland and put her in the psychiatric ward of the hospital and we all flew to her side—my brother and I and even my father—but she remained very confused, laughing one minute, crying the next, raving and incoherent. She wouldn't eat and she wouldn't drink nor would she surrender the fur coat she insisted on wearing in her hospital bed. We thought we'd lost her. But she was a survivor through and through, and three weeks later she was well enough to leave the hospital to convalesce in a clinic. She was a miracle once again, coming back to life from far away.

In her final illness in 2000, even though lovingly cared for by Lorna, her nurse, she no longer had the strength to fight off death or the demons that had always haunted her.

My brother, Philippe, and I buried her in Brussels, beside our father. She knew there was a spot for her there, and was happy about it. They had been each other's big loves in life, even though they separated, and it was appropriate that they end up together. We had our father's headstone engraved: "Thank you for your love," and our mother's: "Thank you for your strength."

The Mullers did not come to the service. Hans had married after they separated and in our agitation after my mother's death, we did not manage to reach his son, Martin, in time for the funeral . . . I feel very bad about that because Martin had remained very close to her; I love him and Lily was a mother to him.

"Today, we're taking Lily, my mother, for her eternal rest," I wrote to her friends and my friends who couldn't be there. "Our hearts are heavy but they should also be light because she has been liberated from all pain and has left on her eternal adventure surrounded by so much love.

"Fifty-five years almost to the day, Lily was liberated from the death camps. Twenty-two years old and less than 28 kilos. In that little package of bones, there was a flame, a flame that was life. Doctors forbade her to have children, she had two. She taught them everything, how to see, question, learn, understand and more important, never to be afraid.

"She touched all the ones that she met, listened to their problems, brought solutions and inspired them to find *joie de vivre* again. She looked so frail and fragile but she was strong and courageous, always curious to discover new horizons. She lived fully and will continue to do so through her children, her grandchildren, her great-grandchildren and her friends who loved her so."

I signed the letter from all of us—"Diane, Philippe, Alexandre, Tatiana, Sarah, Kelly, Talita, and Antonia." (My grandsons Tassilo and Leon were not born yet.)

I found a sweet note among many others my mother had written to herself, had it printed with an embossed lily of the valley because it was her favorite flower, and included it with what I had written.

"God gave me life and luck with my life," she'd written. "During my life, I've kept my luck all along. I have felt it like a shadow. It follows me everywhere and so I take it wherever I go, saying, 'Thank you, my luck. Thank you, my life. Thank you. Thank you.'"

2

LOVE

"Love is life is love is life ..." I first wrote these words inside a heart when asked to design a T-shirt for a charity years ago, in the early nineties. I don't remember which charity it was for, but I do remember taking a photo of the T-shirt on Roffredo Gaetani, an aristocratic, muscular, good-looking Italian ex-boyfriend of mine, cropping his head and turning the photo into a postcard. I still have some of those postcards, and that same drawing marches across my computer screen, has appeared on DVF iPhone cases, canvas shopping bags, graffiti wrap dresses, even babyGap bodysuits. The words from my heart have become my personal mantra and the signature motto for the company.

Love is life is love. There is no way to envision life without love, and at this point in my life, I don't think there is anything more important—love of family, love of nature, love of travel, love of learning, love of life in every way—all of it. Love is being thankful, love is paying attention, love is being open and compassionate. Love is using all the privileges you possess to help those who are in need. Love is giving voice to those who don't have one. Love is a way of feeling alive and respecting life.

I have been in love many times, but I know now that being in love does not always mean you know how to love. Being in love can be a need, a fantasy, or an obsession, whereas loving truly is a much calmer and happier state. I agree with George Sand, the nineteenth-century French novelist: "There is only one happiness in life, to love and be loved," she wrote. I've enjoyed that happiness many times, but what I discovered with age is that true love is unconditional, and that is bliss.

Love is about relationships, yet the most important relationship is the one you have with yourself. Who else is with you at all times? Who else feels the pain when you are hurt? The shame when you are humiliated? Who can smile at your small satisfactions and laugh at your victories but you? Who understands your moments of fear and loneliness better? Who can console you better than you? You are the one who possesses the keys to your being. You carry the passport to your own happiness.

You cannot have a good relationship with anyone, unless you first have it with yourself. Once you have that, any other relationship is a plus, and not a must. "Take time this summer to really get to know yourself," I told a graduating class of high school girls as they were about to start their own journey of life. "Become your best friend; it is well worth it. It takes a lot of work and it can be painful because it requires honesty and discipline. It means you have to accept who you are, see all your faults and weaknesses. Having done that, you can correct, improve, and little by little discover the things you do like about yourself and start to design your life. There is no love un-less there is truth and there is nothing truer than discovering and accepting who you really are. By being critical, you will find things you dislike as well as things you like, and the whole package is who you are. The whole package is what you must embrace and the whole package is what you have control of. It is you! Everything you think, do, like, becomes the person you are and the whole thing weaves into a life, your life."

I finished my talk with an ancient quotation:

> *Beware of your thoughts for they become words,*
> *beware of your words for they become actions,*
> *beware of your actions for they become habits,*
> *beware of your habits for they become character,*
> *beware of your character for it becomes your destiny.*

I was lucky to start a relationship with myself very early in life. I am not sure why; maybe because I had no sibling until the age of six and I was alone a lot, or maybe because I was taught from an early age to be responsible for myself and for my actions.

I remember discovering that little "me" person in the reflection of my mother's vanity mirror and being intrigued by it. Not that I loved my image, but as I made funny and ugly faces at my own reflection, I enjoyed the control I had over it; I could make it do anything I wanted. I was absorbed by that little "me" person and wanted to discover more about her. Later, when I learned to write, I wrote stories about this character and the fantasies I imagined for her. The fictional stories became rarer as I turned to writing my diaries, recounting my experiences, my frustrations, my sense of cosmic emptiness, or my desire to conquer. My diary became my friend, my refuge.

My teenage diaries got lost and though I wish I still had them,

I rarely look back at the ones I do have. Their importance was in the moment, of having a friend to confide in. At this point in my life, I seldom write in my diaries. I have replaced the writing with a visual diary. I carry a camera with me everywhere and take pictures of what I want to store in my memory—people, nature, objects, architecture. Often I use those photos for inspiration.

I also learned how critical it is for me to have time alone to recharge and strengthen that inner connection. It is easy to lose oneself when you are with people all the time. I need silence and solitude to create a buffer against the daily barrage of information and challenges. Sometimes, in a big crowd, even at parties that I host, I find myself disappearing for a few minutes to be alone. I used to feel sad and out of place in those moments, lonely and disconnected. I don't anymore. I use these moments to reconnect with myself and build my strength.

Equally soothing and crucial is my love and need for nature. Nothing is more nourishing than seeing the day appear from the night, the strength of the waves, the majesty of the trees. Walking in the woods, being lost in nature reminds me of how small we are in the universe and somehow that reassures me. I remember one day walking in the country with my then very small son, Alexandre. I was lost in thought and when he inquired what those thoughts were, I responded, "I wonder what will happen to us." Very wisely little Alexandre answered, "I know what will happen, Mommy. Spring will come and the leaves will cover the trees again, then it will be summer, then autumn and the leaves will change color and fall. Winter and snow will follow." I smiled and took his hand. "Of course that is what will happen," I answered. I never forgot that moment.

Love is life is love and like most mothers, my strongest love has always been for my children. I'll never forget the intense rush I felt the first time I saw Alexandre. Not only was he my firstborn, I felt as if I already knew him. I had had many long conversations with him before he was born and I have always felt he was my partner as much as my son.

Alexandre was also the answer to my dream as a young girl—to have a little American son when I grew up. As a European girl, I always thought American boys were cooler, more casual and more boyish. Boys in Europe seemed serious and sometimes even repressed and I loved that American boys, who watched football and played sports endlessly, were not. Anyway, I got exactly what I wanted: a real little American boy, though he carries Egon's title of "prince." However, as I've watched the grown Alexandre raise his own American boys, I've realized that I failed him at least in one thing—I did not pay enough attention to his athletic life and seldom went to his games when he was growing up. I was never the Soccer Mom he secretly wished for.

In many respects I didn't know what I was doing when he was a baby, because, like any young mother, I had no experience. I was a little intimidated and relied heavily on our Italian nanny until I happened upon her handling Alexandre roughly in the bath—and fired her. From then on, no longer intimidated, I followed my common sense.

Beautiful, mischievous Princess Tatiana Desiree von und zu Furstenberg followed her brother thirteen months later. She was something else. I said from the beginning that she was the drop of oil you put into egg yolks and mustard to make mayonnaise happen. She was the magic that turned we three into a real family. When Tatiana was born, it wasn't Egon and me having a child, it was Egon, Alexandre, and me becoming a full family. And though the marriage didn't last, we remained a family forever.

I have great empathy with working mothers and the tug of war they feel, as I did, between staying with my children and going off to work. It never occurred to me to give up my growing business because I insisted on paying all my bills and took no money from Egon when we separated, but it was always wrenching to walk out the door. Once outside, however, I felt free, energized, and focused on making a good life for all of us. And it quickly came true all because of that little wrap dress.

With the first money I earned, I bought Cloudwalk, an astonishingly beautiful property in Connecticut for my twenty-seventh birthday so we could spend relaxed time together in a setting where we could also feel free. And we did. I spent much time there with the children and their school friends, cooking for them and often transporting one of them to the emergency room to see if a cut needed stitches or an arm was more than just bruised. During the week I'd be a tycooness in New York again, striding out the door in my high heels and fishnet stockings. I winked in the mirror, smiled at my shadow, and off I went, to make a living and become the woman I wanted to be.

From the beginning, I treated Alexandre and Tatiana more as people than as children. I never talked down to them and always encouraged them to express their opinions and take responsibility for themselves. Making me independent is what my mother did for me, and I was, for sure, going to do that for my children. Just as I had started keeping a journal in my childhood, I urged them to start recording their lives and thoughts. They began even before they were old enough to read and write, drawing the events of their days in pictures. We ended the day by exchanging news about what they'd done at school and what I'd done at work during "discussion time" on their beds. I involved them in every facet of my life, including my business.

"I have my job and school is your job," I told them. "We all go to work, we all have our own lives, we all have our responsibilities. You deliver on yours and I'll deliver on mine." It turned out to be a very good approach. Tatiana excelled at school, Alex did very well, and I managed all right at work.

I took them with me on trips as often as I could and, in spite of themselves, they became very good travelers. They would often complain or be upset about traveling conditions that seemed dangerous or boring to them at the moment, but those moments from their unusual adventures ended up being wonderful memories and great stories to tell. I remember a trip to the very isolated, prehistoric island of Nias across from Sumatra in the Indonesian archipelago. The tiny little local boat we took was fragile, to say the least. The return crossing in the middle of the night was rough, hot, and buggy. We kept silent as I prayed that we would make it safely to the mainland. Exotic it was, but maybe too exotic, risky, and dangerous, but we made it. That trip ended up in both their college applications in answer to the question: "What was one of the most riveting and adventurous things you've done in your life?"

In such extreme circumstances, and in other, calmer ones, I treasured traveling with my children. Traveling with children is unique because it is about discovering together. You are equal in front of new things and experiences. I always found it a great period of closeness, and I recommend it to parents. You lose the power role a bit and become companions. You don't have to say look at this and look at that because you're discovering at the same time—the landscapes you see, the people you encounter, the lines for tickets, the stop for lunch, the unexpected.

Could I have become the woman I wanted to be without having children? I certainly would not have been the same person. In fact, it's very hard, impossible really, for me to imagine what my life would have been without them. We actually grew up together. I was twenty-four when I had them both, barely a grown-up myself. I wasn't old enough to have yearned for children, yet suddenly there they were and my responsibility. I loved them with an intensity I'd never felt before. They were a part of me forever.

I was helped enormously by their two amazing grandmothers, both of whom were very present in my children's lives. My mother came to live with us in New York for months during the school year and struck her own loving relationship with them. Egon's mother, Clara Agnelli Nuvoletti, was just as attentive. The children spent almost every vacation with her, either on the island of Capri, at her house outside Venice, or in the mountain chalet in Cortina. My mother had become a very good friend of Clara's, and often she went along so my children had two fantastic grandmothers with them.

How wonderful it was, especially for Tatiana. Alexandre started going off on various adventures like glacier skiing and sailing, but Tatiana preferred staying with her grandmothers. She learned French from my mother and Italian and cooking from Clara. Her second husband, Giovanni Nuvoletti, was the president of the culinary academy of Italy and Clara wrote several cookbooks. Tatiana became an excellent cook and often cooks for us now. She also had long philosophical discussions with both of her grandmothers about love and the meaning of life. Clara would make her laugh with the gossip of her very privileged life and my mother would remind her of the challenges of adversity.

Unlike me, the grandmothers had nothing but time, which was wonderful for the children and wonderful for me. They had such a strong and very important influence: They were teachers, role models, active participants, and, above all, loving family members. Both had memories to share, both had great senses of humor, and both were great storytellers.

In a house with three women—my mother, Tatiana, and me—Alexandre was always considered the man of the house. He was the one we trained to be counted on. Now that he is a grown man, he has become all the things I had wished him to be. He watches over our assets and has become very valuable to the growth of DVF. Tatiana also became an important protector of the family: a specialist in diagnosing illnesses and best at giving advice. Now they both watch over Barry and me. We all sit on the board of DVF and we share the Diller–von Furstenberg Family Foundation. My children are the bookends that support me. We talk on the phone every day, sometimes more than once. "I love you," "I love you, too," we end each conversation.

If I have one regret in my life, it is that I didn't pay more attention to Tatiana when, in fact, she was the one who needed it more. In contrast to Alexandre, who was quite a wild boy and reduced me to pleading tears when he became a very fast teenage driver, Tatiana was such a good girl and caused so few problems that I took her for granted. This was a mistake. I didn't realize until much later that because she so rarely did anything to draw attention to herself, she felt I cared less about her than I did her brother. That brought an ache to my heart because I love them both with equal intensity, but I could see how she felt that way. Alexandre did get more of my attention because Tatiana didn't seem to need it. I was completely wrong.

From the time she could walk, Tatiana's legs seemed quite stiff. She could certainly get around all right, but she was never able to run. Her condition grew more noticeable when she began school and had difficulty with sports. I took her to several orthopedists, who checked her bones and looked to see if she had scoliosis, but they said there was nothing the matter with her, that her muscles were just stiffer than others and she would probably grow out of it. She didn't. Instead she hid her suffering from all of us for years until one day in her early twenties when she tried to run across Park Avenue and collapsed on the pavement. What a wrenching sight she was with two black eyes and a hugely swollen lip because she couldn't raise her arms in time to block her fall. Tatiana had just completed her master's degree in psychology at the time and remembered a reference to neuromuscular disorders. A neurologist at Columbia Presbyterian finally gave her a diagnosis: myotonia, a genetic muscular disorder that delays the muscles from relaxing after any exercise, especially in cold weather.

"Why didn't your mother know this before?" the doctor asked in wonderment, a question that stabbed my heart. We'd been going to orthopedists, who were concerned only with her bones.

I felt awful for her and angry at myself. When we'd first tried to address her condition she was at Spence School in New York, where she and the other girls in the Lower School had to walk up and down nine flights of stairs several times a day. What agony it must have been for her, but I didn't know about it because she never complained. Her suffering only increased when I moved the children to Cloudwalk, our house in Connecticut, when she was in the fifth grade, and the school there stressed athletics. Tatiana struggled and struggled, thinking her disability was all in her head—one doctor had told her flat out there was nothing wrong with her—but still, she didn't complain. Like my mother, Tatiana refused to think of herself as a victim.

I will never forgive myself for not realizing or understanding the scope of her disability, how it made her feel different from the other children and was a source of great physical and emotional pain. We have since had many long, long conversations about it, and I discovered that, just as I hadn't wanted to upset my mother, she didn't want to worry me when she was growing up. She saw the pressure and stress I was under with my business (she and Alexandre always called my business my "third child") and she didn't want to add any more pressure on me.

In 2014, Tatiana learned she does not have myotonia, but rather Brody disease, also a genetic condition that affects the muscles, including the muscle of the heart, which further explains her difficulty to keep pace with others. It brought home again how difficult it has been for her all her life. I wish she had told me. But maybe she did and I just did not hear it. I have kept a little note from her that she wrote to me as a very small child. It is on the bulletin board in my office in Cloudwalk. I cherished that note because I thought it was so sweet. It said "Mommy, you really know nothing about me." How awful I feel today when I look at this note that I thought was so sweet, and neither she nor I understood that it was a cry for help.

Tatiana may not be able to move as fast as everyone else, but her intelligence, her imagination, her heart, and her talent are so immense that she will continue to realize all of her dreams.

Tatiana always got the best grades in school—she was summa cum laude at her school in Connecticut—and did so well that she skipped the seventh grade. She always did her brother's homework as well as her own and held it over him for years, constantly reminding Alexandre: "I did your homework for you. I did your applications for you and I did your thesis for you," but she also admits that now she's getting paid back by Alexandre through his financial skills.

Tatiana never much liked the schools she went to so she just kept on jumping— from day school in Connecticut, to a year at boarding school in Switzerland, another in England, and then to Brown University at the age of sixteen. She graduated in just over three years. I was so very, very proud of her. I went to her graduation along with my mother and Mila, my housekeeper from France who had been very close to Tatiana, and was touched beyond measure when she presented me with a bouquet of flowers in gratitude for all I'd done for her. But even better than the flowers, I loved watching her huge smile and incredible beauty on that victorious day. Alexandre went to Brown, too, and graduated a year after Tatiana (though he is a year older) so both my children are better educated than I am.

I feel more and more connected to both children as the years go by. I can usually feel when something is wrong and when they need me. For me it is always "us," never "I." And that will never change. I look at them now, and love them, respect them, and admire them. Alex, an exceptional father, lover of life, and brilliant businessman and asset manager. Tatiana, a wonderful mother, a certified teacher and therapist, and a successful screenwriter and director. Her first feature film, *Tanner Hall*, which she cowrote, directed, and produced with her friend Francesca Gregorini, was the winner of the 2011 GENART Film Festival Audience Award, and launched Rooney Mara from her first starring role to a Best Actress Oscar nomination for *The Girl with the Dragon Tattoo*.

I like to joke that the children are my best samples, but those samples are definitely not for sale. As I look at them as adults and almost-beginning-to-age adults, it is possible for me to claim both success and failure in the kind of mother I was. I couldn't do that at the beginning of their lives, and certainly not during their teenage years when my constant prayer was to get them through it alive. But now I can enjoy the harvest from the seeds planted so many years ago and relax a little—though not too much.

The greatest thing about becoming a grandparent is watching your children being parents. For the first time you realize that they actually heard the things you told them throughout their childhoods. I see it in the way they make their children independent, the way they give them freedom, push them to make their own decisions, love and support them.

Just as my mother annoyed me with endless advice, I am sure I annoyed my children passing on that advice and a lot of my own, but it has paid off with my grandchildren. Alexandre's oldest child, Talita, the firstborn and now a teenager, is very much like her father, so I have a tendency to be both demanding and to take her for granted. She is beautiful and very bright, a great debater, a talented painter, and has an old soul. We love to talk about everything—the business of DVF, my mother's experience during the war, politics—everything. When she was nine I took her with me to Florence where I was preparing a fashion show in the private garden of a beautiful mansion. "Do you want to come with me and be my assistant?" I asked her. "I'm going to be working so you will have to work, too." "Yes, yes," she said, and she took part in all the magic of preparing a fashion show—watching the sets being made, casting the models, doing the fittings, choosing the final looks. We had a delightful and unforgettable week, stealing time out during the day to go to museums and at night to watch romantic comedies set in Europe like *Funny Face* and *Sabrina* from the Audrey Hepburn collection I had brought along.

When Talita's younger brother Tassilo was ten, Barry and I took him to the 2012 Olympics in London. At first I was a bit concerned what I would do alone with a little boy, but we ended up having a great time watching basketball and volleyball and laughing all the way. Tassilo is named for Egon's father, Prince Tassilo Egon Maximilian—and he was born very much a little prince, a little American prince. I don't really know what I mean by that, but that's the way we all look at him. He is cool, cute, and very kind, an excellent athlete and a good student. "I like to chill" is the way he describes himself.

Antonia, Tatiana's daughter, is a star. I think of her as the militant in the family, the political person, an A student, compassionate, a good painter, a born performer, and an amazing musician. She can hear a song and immediately play it on the piano. She impressed everyone at one of the DVF Christmas talent shows when, at the age of eleven, she performed an Adele song, not as a child but as a true artist. She is also wonderfully strong and centered. I got an indignant email from her after I sent a "Happy International Women's Day" email. "Shouldn't it be women's and girls' day?" she emailed me. "Aren't we women, too?"

Antonia, who, like me and her mother, went to boarding school in England, is great company. I have spent wonderful days alone with her in New York, London, Paris, and Shanghai, where we stole a day to visit the small towns outside the city known for their gorgeous gardens.

Barry and I spend every Christmas and New Year's holiday with the grandchildren, sometimes on our boat, other times on a land adventure. Since my birthday is on New Year's Eve, I always get a surprise from them: a collage, a song they have written, or a birthday cake in bed, as I remember from a wonderful New Year's holiday in Patagonia, Chile. And letters. We always exchange New Year's letters full of love and good wishes.

All grandparents think their grandchildren are amazing and I am biased, no doubt. As I write, I am recently blessed with a fourth grandchild, Leon (named for my father). It is Alexandre's third child and his first with AK, as we call his beautiful love and life companion, Alison Kay. I look forward to having a special relationship with little Leon as I have with the others.

I have loved a lot and have been in love many, many times. Perhaps I've been in love so often because I asked little in return or maybe because I was just in love with being in love. For me, falling in love wasn't a need—it was an adventure. My father so filled me with love that I didn't think I needed, or wanted, much back. That emotional independence made some men feel insecure and frustrated, and others relieved. Not that I was never like every girl, dependent or jealous at times, waiting for "the" phone call or behaving stupidly. Of course I did, many, many times.

The first time I remember being in love was with a boy in Brussels who had absolutely no interest in me. His name was Charlie Bouchonville. I would see him in the NR4 tramway coming home from school. He had green eyes and a beauty spot at the end of his left eye, wore a suede jacket, and was very stylish. I was still a little girl, flat chested and all. I don't think he ever knew I existed, but I fantasized about him for a long time, and when I went to boarding school I boasted about a relationship with him that had never existed.

The first boy I kissed was Italian. His name was Vanni, short for Giovanni, and we kissed in the tearoom of the Hotel Rouge in Milano Marittima where my mother, brother, and I were spending a holiday on the Adriatic coast of Italy. I was fourteen. Vanni was a very, very sexy boy, who must have been more than eighteen because he was proudly driving a little yellow Alfa Romeo. We would meet after lunch in the tearoom of the hotel and kiss. My mother would send Philippe as a spy and he would just sit there. Philippe and I were sharing a bedroom and one night Vanni snuck up to our room while my brother was sleeping. I felt very grown up in the midst of our whispers and tiptoeing around the room, but I disappointed Vanni. He wanted to do more than I was willing to do, so our lovely flirtation stayed pretty much at the kissing level. We wrote letters to each other for a while afterward, which was perfect for my Italian. I learned Italian writing love letters.

My first serious boyfriend was called Sohrab. He was born in Iran and was studying architecture in Oxford. He had a beautiful smile, drove a turquoise Volkswagen, and was very nice to me. I had just arrived at Stroud Court, a boarding school for girls outside Oxford. School had not started but I had come early, as had Danae, a Greek girl from Athens who became my best friend that year. Danae and I went to see an exhibition of Henry Moore sculptures at the Ashmolean Museum, and afterward we went for tea across the street at the Randolph Hotel. There we met these two cute Persian boys, Sohrab and Shidan, and we immediately became great friends.

Our school allowed us to go out on Wednesday afternoons, all day Saturday, and Sunday afternoons. The next Wednesday, Sohrab took me to the movies to see *Dr. No*, the first James Bond. I could hardly follow the dialogue because my English was not very good, but I had a wonderful afternoon. Sohrab was kind and thoughtful. My parents were going through an unpleasant divorce, and the letters I received from home made me feel powerless and sad. Sohrab consoled me and took me to eat Indian food. I had never been in a restaurant with a boy before and it felt very special.

Later we would go to his room on Banbury Road. All he had was a large desk by the window and a big bed. It was very cold and humid and every hour he would put a sixpence coin into the heater to keep it going. His bed was cozy and so was he. We kissed a lot. I was a virgin and was still wearing little girl cotton underwear, which I felt embarrassed about. I wanted to pretend I was older and sophisticated but I did not really want to have sex. We broke up for a while and then started seeing each other again. By then I had bought silk underwear. I was sixteen. He became my first lover, kind and attentive. He made me happy. Many, many years later I found out that I, too, was his first lover. He was twenty-one.

The following summer, I was on holiday in Riccione, Italy, with my father and brother. Sohrab and Shidan drove from England to see me on their way to Iran, where they were going to sell the little turquoise Volkswagen for a profit before going back to Oxford. They did not stay long, barely an afternoon. To this day, my brother, who was still a child, remembers and doesn't understand what happened next. One day I was clearly in love with Sohrab, keeping his framed photo by my bed in my hotel room. The next day, I met Lucio on the beach. He became my next boyfriend.

Lucio was a very handsome twenty-two-year-old who looked like the Italian actor Marcello Mastroianni. We fell in love. He was passionate and experienced. He would hold my arm firmly and take me into the pine forest behind the beach. He would make love to me endlessly, making me feel like a real woman. During the day I was a normal seventeen-year-old girl having a nice holiday with her father and brother, but at night I had a secret life, a grown-up woman having a very sexy love affair. Lucio was very much in love and so was I.

We kept up a passionate correspondence for a long time and every now and then would manage to meet. Once, in Milan, where I had accompanied my father on a business trip, we locked ourselves in a hotel room near the railroad station for the entire day. Another time I went to Crevalcore near Bologna where he lived. Taking advantage of the fact that my mother was on a trip with Hans, I left boarding school early and took a detour to Italy on the way home to Geneva. I met his family, who had a small handbag factory. They organized a dinner for me in a local restaurant and I slept in a tiny hotel near his home. Later on he came twice to visit me while I was studying in Spain. Our passionate encounters remain a wild memory.

Two years ago I received a sad letter from Lucio's wife. He had died and she had found letters from me and some photographs. Would I like to have them? "Of course," I said, and to my delight I received a huge box with hundreds of love letters I had sent him as well as photos, menus, and train tickets. He had kept them all.

In England after the holiday I became infatuated with a French girl at my school. Her name was Deanna. She was very shy and masculine and she intrigued me. We became very close. We went on together to the University of Madrid where there were so many anti-Franco riots and so many strikes that we hardly ever went to class as the university was almost always closed. We shared a grim little room in a pensione for girls on the Calle de la Libertad in the center of Madrid. To get into our pensione at night, we had to clap and the Serrano, who held the keys for the block, would open our building's door and let us in. We made friends at the Facultad de Filosofía y Letras where we took Estudios Hispánicos classes. We watched flamencos at night and went to bullfights on Sundays. Madrid was a repressed city at the time, still wounded from the civil war. The mood was dark and I was bored.

My life took a different turn during the Christmas holiday that year. My mother, Hans, his son Martin, my brother, and I went to celebrate the holidays in Gstaad in the Swiss Alps. We were staying at the Hôtel du Parc having a dull time when suddenly, one afternoon in the village, I bumped into my best friend from Pensionnat Cuche, my boarding school in Lausanne. Isabel was from Venezuela, a bit older than I, beautiful and sophisticated. It was Isabel who had taught me how to French-kiss, practicing on mirrors. She lived with her mother and sister in Paris; her father, Juan Liscano, was a famous writer and intellectual in Caracas.

The encounter with Isabel changed the course of my life because that night she took me to a party and I made my official entry into the jet set world. The party was at the chalet of the Shorto family, a Brazilian/English lady and her five gorgeous children. The music was loud, people were dancing samba, smoking, drinking, laughing, and speaking many languages at the same time. Everyone seemed to know each other. I had never experienced that atmosphere before. They took me in immediately. I became part of the group and stayed on with Isabel after my family went back home to Geneva.

In Gstaad I met an "older man" in his midthirties who took a liking to me and never left my side for a week. His name was Vlady Blatnik. He lived in Venezuela where he had a successful shoe business. Vlady took me to dinner parties and we went skiing together every day. For New Year's Eve, my birthday, he bought me a Pucci printed silk top with black silk pants and matching black silk boots. This was my first designer outfit. That night I turned nineteen and even though I did not feel as beautiful or glamorous as the other women in the room, I thought life had finally begun!

Going back to Madrid to complete the school year was a bit of a downer, but during spring break Deanna and I planned a trip through Andalusia. We discovered the beauty of the Alhambra in Grenada and the magic of Sevilla. That trip was the end of my stay in Spain. I decided to continue school in Geneva where my mother was living with Hans. Deanna moved to Andalusia, and we stayed friends for a bit then lost touch.

I called Deanna a few years ago to invite her to the opening of my new boutique in Honolulu where she now lives. We picked up where we left off, as childhood friends do. "Can you believe we are in our sixties?" I said. We laughed at the absurdity of it. I felt the same age I was when I last saw her.

I have always tried to stay in touch with the people that were important in my life and the people that I loved. Once I love, I love forever, and there is nothing more cozy and meaningful than old friends and lovers. I'm so fortunate to have had and have so much love in my life. Without it, I would never be who I am.

I find great happiness in my relationships with old friends, living mirrors that reflect histories of laughter and sorrow, triumphs and failures, births and deaths, on both sides.

My closest, oldest friend is Olivier Gelbsmann, who has known me since I was eighteen. He has followed every step of my life and when we are together we don't need to speak to know what the other thinks. Olivier worked with me very early on, worked with Egon afterward, and later became an interior decorator. We now work together on DVF décor and home products. Olivier was present when my children were born, and at every important moment of my life. He consoled each of my boyfriends when I left them. Olivier was friends with my mother, my daughter, and now my granddaughters. My friend the Greek artist Konstantin Kakanias, with whom I collaborated on an inspirational comic book, *Be the Wonder Woman You Can Be,* as well as other projects, has also been friends with four generations of women in my family.

I treasure the memories I share with friends like Olivier and Konstantin. Landscapes change, people come and go, but all the landscapes, all the experiences, all the people weave into your life's fabric. Love is not just about people you had affairs with. Love is about moments of intimacy, paying attention to others, connecting. As you learn that love is everywhere, you find it everywhere.

Just as I collect books and textiles, I collect memories and friends. I love to remember. It's not that I dwell in nostalgia, but that I love intimacy. It is the opposite of small talk. It is the closest thing to truth.

"Beauty is truth, truth beauty," as I learned in Oxford when I studied the English poet John Keats.

I have tried not to lie my whole life. Lies are toxic. They are the beginning of misunderstandings, complications, and unhappiness. To practice truth is not always easy, but as with all practices, it becomes a matter of habit. Truth is cathartic, a way of keeping the trees pruned. The truer you can be the better it is because it simplifies life and love.

––––––––––

There are many degrees of love, of course. I know now that of all the so many times I've been in love, only two men were truly great loves. I married both of them, one toward the beginning of my life, the other much later.

Egon. I cannot begin to describe all I owe to my first husband, Prince Eduard Egon von und zu Fürstenberg. I will be forever thankful to him because he gave me so much. He gave me my children; he gave me his name; he gave me his trust and his encouragement as he believed in me; he shared everything, all of his knowledge and all of his connections as he gave me his love.

I met Egon at a birthday party in Lausanne. I remember his big smile, his childlike face, and his gapped teeth. He had just enrolled at the University of Geneva where I was taking courses. He had also just returned from a few months in a Catholic mission in Burundi, where he had taught children and taken care of leprosy patients. I was impressed. I remember what I was wearing the night I met him because he complimented me on it—pink palazzo pajama pants and an embroidered tunic I had borrowed from my mother's closet. We were both nineteen.

Egon was the perfect eligible bachelor, an Austro/German prince by his father, and a rich heir from his mother, Clara Agnelli, the eldest child of the Fiat motorcar family. Egon seemed interested in me, maybe because I had already made a lot of friends in Geneva, and he had just arrived. We went out a lot and one Sunday we drove to nearby Megève in the mountains for a day in the snow. The car broke down and Egon went to get help. I remember opening the glove compartment to check his passport. I had never met a prince before and I wanted to see if his title was written on it. (It was not). When Egon came back to the car with a mechanic, the engine started immediately. There was nothing wrong with the car. To this day I remember Egon's embarrassed face. It was his helplessness that seduced me.

Egon lived in a small, luxurious rental apartment near Lac Léman while I was living at home with my mother and Hans, but we were always together. My mother, who had never acknowledged a boyfriend of mine before, immediately adopted him. They would become very close. Egon had a lot of energy and a great sense of adventure. He was always planning trips and places to discover. He suggested a group of us join a package deal trip to the Far East. I managed to convince my mother to let me go with them only for her to discover when she brought me to the airport that the only passengers going were Egon and me. The others had dropped out. I panicked, worried she wouldn't let me go alone with Egon, but she did.

We had a great time. India, New Delhi, Agra, and the magnificent Taj Mahal, Thailand and its floating market, Burma and its hundred pagodas, Cambodia and the ruins of Angkor Wat, the making of clothes overnight in Hong Kong. We went sightseeing all day every day as perfect tourists, and at night, we were invited to dine with local people through Egon's Fiat connection. Egon was the most charming young man in the world. His charisma and enthusiasm were contagious and traveling with him was always full of surprises and serendipity.

In Bangkok we dined with Jim Thompson, a famous American who had settled in Thailand after the war and had organized all the independent silk weavers into the huge business he owned, the Thai Silk Company. Mr. Thompson was wearing a silk shirt and pants and embroidered velvet slippers. He lived in a magnificent old Thai house full of antiques. From the house, we could see the weavers working at night, lit by lanterns, all along the floating market. I remember him telling us he was leaving for a holiday the next day in the jungles of Malaysia. He was never to be seen again. Rumors say that he was a double, triple agent and had been killed.

Another night, in Thailand, I was so mad at Egon—I'd found him in our hotel room having a massage from a beautiful Thai girl—that I'd gone down to the bar. A rather gloomy American man bought me a very strong Thai beer, announced he worked for a defense contractor, then said, "Oh well, the Vietnam War will soon be finished, but it doesn't matter because there will be a new arms market now in the Middle East." (Two months later, the 1967 Six-Day War erupted in Israel, Jordan, and Syria.) I was shocked. I had never realized that wars actually meant business for some people. They use research, marketing, sales—everything a normal company does—but for the business of weapons and war. It was a jolt to learn that as soon as defense contractors hear there is a conflict somewhere, they send salesmen and open a new market.

Egon and I went everywhere and discovered everything together. I remember the first time he took me to Villa Bella, his mother's chalet in Cortina d'Ampezzo in the Italian Alps. I had never been in such an elegant, welcoming, unusual house before. All in wood, it looked like a glorified gingerbread house full of antiques, an unexpected mix of colorful fabrics and quantities of silver and Murano glass. There were many housemaids dressed in Tyrolean fashion and butlers in full gear, yet the household was not stiff. The young ones would go skiing all day and gather with all the others for dinner. Food was abundant and delicious, of course, and the conversation humorous and superficial.

Clara, Egon's mother, was there with Count Giovanni Nuvoletti, who was to become her second husband a few years later. Giovanni was a writer and a man of the salon. He was very eloquent and held court, while Clara was light and witty. We were a group of friends from university who had come to Villa Bella for the Christmas holidays, and I shared a room with a beautiful redheaded girl called Sandy. I celebrated my twentieth birthday there, still feeling slightly out of place. By the time I celebrated my twenty-first birthday in that same villa the following year, I had become more comfortable and at ease with the family, the milieu, the lifestyle in general.

Egon took me to the South of France to meet his glamorous uncle Gianni Agnelli on his yacht and to watch the Grand Prix of Monaco, the famous car race. He took me to the film festival at the Lido of Venice and the Volpi Ball on the Canale Grande. I met everyone that was anyone anywhere—aristocrats, courtesans, businesspeople, actors, painters, and all of the Café Society entourage. How would I ever remember all these names, places, all this information, I wondered, taken by the dizziness of it all. It all felt like what Hemingway so eloquently described as a "moveable feast."

But our experiences were not only about glamour and wealth. Egon was a real traveler, inquisitive, full of energy and curiosity, eager to meet all kinds of people in whatever country we were in, keen to eat into the adventure—sometimes literally. I remember a man he befriended in the old souks of Djerba, Tunisia, who invited us to his house for lunch. We followed him through the narrow twisting alleyways, turning to the left, to the right, and to the left again, having no idea where we were going. We finally arrived in what looked like an abandoned apartment building, climbed the stairs, and arrived in the man's house, filled with children, some of whom were obviously sick. Food was served and I couldn't touch it, I felt repulsed, but Egon downed it with grace as if we were at the most elegant home in Paris. I will always remember that day, the lesson it taught me. Egon had an incredible ease about him, which made all people feel good about themselves. He was a true prince.

I'd traveled a lot with my family as a child, but Egon brought it to a different level. He infused in me the same curiosity and sense of adventure, which I carry to this day. I'm always ready to go. I pack lightly. I travel lightly, leaving time for the unknown. Even as a child I loved to travel, through my Tintin books. It was with Tintin that I learned geography and discovered the world first—America, Egypt, Peru, China, the Congo. When I arrive somewhere I have never been before, I always think of Tintin.

But Egon's most important gift was our children, all the more because I was hesitant about having them, especially Alexandre. He was the unexpected result of a weekend I spent with Egon in Rome in May 1969. I was living in Italy then, working as an intern for a fashion industrialist, Angelo Ferretti. Egon was taking the summer off, having completed his training program at Chase Manhattan Bank in New York, and was on his way to India and the Far East with a friend from school, Marc Landeau, before starting another job at the investment bank Lazard Frères in New York. I was very excited to see him and he, evidently, me. He had organized a big dinner with friends at Tula, a fashionable restaurant off Via Condotti, and I went with him wearing an evening jumpsuit with a plunging décolleté we had bought on sale that afternoon on the Via Gregoriana.

I remember there were paparazzi outside in the streets, but what happened inside was brighter than all of their flashbulbs. Egon gave me a beautiful ring he had designed, a pale sapphire in a big gold setting. To my complete surprise, this dinner was an engagement party. I was very excited, even though I did not totally believe it. Yet that night, in the intimacy of our bedroom, I remember whispering to Egon: "I will give you a son." Did I really mean it? Or was I only trying to be seductive? In any event, after the weekend, Egon went to India and I went back to Ferretti's factory.

A few weekends later I went to Monaco with friends to watch the Grand Prix again. Ferretti was in Monaco, too, and offered me a ride back to Milan at the end of the weekend. He drove his Maserati very fast and I thought it was all the high-speed twists and turns in the road that were making me nauseated. I felt even more sick the next day and thought a sauna might make me feel better. It didn't. Instead I fainted in the middle of Piazza San Babila and remember hearing people saying "She's dead, she's dead" and all I could do was move a finger to show them "No, I'm not dead." What I was, of course, was pregnant. I couldn't believe my ears when the doctor told me the news.

Here I was, barely twenty-two, and what I wanted most was to be independent. Furthermore, Egon was one of the best "catches" in Europe. Who was going to believe that I had not done it on purpose? I went home to Geneva to see another doctor who told me he could help me end the pregnancy. I was torn.

I went to my mother for advice. She had taken Egon's gift of a ring more seriously than I had and was horrified at the thought that I could make such a decision on my own. "You are engaged," she said. "The least you can do is discuss the matter with your fiancé."

Reluctantly, I drafted a telegram to Egon, who was in Hong Kong, offering him the choice. I have kept the telegram of his wonderful reply in my scrapbook. He was clear and definite. "Only one option. Organize marriage in Paris July 15. I rejoice. Thinking of you. Love and kisses, Eduard Egon."

Suddenly my life was giving me vertigo, though it was a happy dizziness. No time to waste. All the wedding preparations: invitations to be printed, wedding dress to be made, ceremony and party to be arranged, trousseau to be bought. As usual, my mother was a great help. We visited Clara, Egon's mother, in Venice and planned it all together.

Clara was very supportive, but on Egon's father's side, the patriarch of the Furstenberg family was evidently not. Jewish blood in the family was unheard of and there was opposition. I also overheard a slight at the Agnelli house—something I interpreted as a clever, ambitious little bourgeois girl from Belgium getting what she wanted. I felt belittled and hurt and remember walking with a very determined stride around Clara's garden, caressing my pregnant stomach. It was then I had my first conversation with Alexandre. "We'll show them," I said out loud to my unborn child. "We'll show them who we are!"

The wedding took place on July 16, 1969, the same day that the first American astronauts were sent to the moon, in the countryside outside Paris, in Montfort l'Amaury. My three-month pregnancy did not show at all in the Christian Dior wedding dress its designer Mark Bohan had created for me. The mayor married us at the town hall and there was a huge luncheon reception afterward at the Auberge de la Moutière, a charming inn and restaurant managed by Maxim's.

The crowd was young, beautiful, and glamorous; the food exquisite; and the entertainment enthusiastic. My father had hired the entire company of fifty musicians and singers from the trendy Russian night-club Raspoutine. To my embarrassment, he took the microphone, sang in Russian with the Raspoutine musicians, and broke glasses. Everyone else loved it and the wedding party was a huge success. The only nonparticipant was Egon's father, Tassilo, who had been so pressured by the family's disapproving patriarch that he came to the ceremony but boycotted the reception, though it barely diminished the celebration or our joy. Egon and I left the guests dancing and singing, and went back to the center of Paris, changed our clothes, and went walking the streets and in an out of the shops of the Faubourg St-Honoré.

For our wedding present his mother gave us a beach house on Sardinia's beautiful Costa Smeralda, where for the whole month of August we packed a crowd of sixteen friends into three tiny bedrooms. We were all so young and had so much fun.

Our beautiful son, Alexandre Egon, was born six months later on January 25, 1970, in New York. Our equally beautiful daughter, Tatiana Desirée, followed just thirteen months later. Just as Egon insisted that we marry and have Alexandre, he was insistent that I have Tatiana. I'd gotten pregnant again just three months after the very difficult birth of Alexandre by emergency cesarean after sixteen hours of labor. The idea of starting all over again needed some encouragement. Lovely Tatiana was born on February 16, 1971, this time by a scheduled cesarean. There are no words to describe how grateful I am for Egon's enthusiasm and support. He played a bigger part in both my children being born than I did, though I played a bigger part afterward.

———————

Life in New York was lots of fun in the early seventies. Real estate was cheap, so many diverse and creative people could live there.

Pop art in the galleries and nudity on Broadway made us feel that everything was new, allowed, and the freedom we felt had just been invented. Prince and Princess von Furstenberg (we had dropped the "und zu") were the "it" couple in town. Our youth, our looks, and our means put us on every invitation list and in social columns. On any given night, we went out to at least one cocktail party, a dinner, sometimes a ball, and always a stop at some gay bar at the end of the night. We lived on Park Avenue but still felt very European and continued to spend a lot of time there.

We hosted lots of parties for Europeans coming to town. I remember the big party we gave for Yves Saint Laurent and the last-minute dinner we gave for Bernardo Bertolucci, who had just opened *Last Tango in Paris*. The movie was quite racy and shocking and its talented and handsome director was the hit of New York. Everyone came to our parties—Andy Warhol and his entourage, actors, designers, journalists, and, of course, many Europeans. Life was fast, to say the least, too fast, finally, for me.

The marriage itself had its own stresses. Egon was my husband and my first true love, but our marriage became complicated. He loved to have fun and was very promiscuous, wanting to experiment as much as possible. I tried to embrace his behavior and accept an open marriage; I certainly did not want to judge him. I acted cool and hid my suffering, not wanting to be a victim. But I had two young children to take care of and was starting an equally demanding business. It finally became too hard to manage it all.

Strangely enough, what saved our relationship and preserved our love was the end of our marriage in 1973. The tipping point was a February cover story about us in *New York* magazine: "The Couple Who

Has Everything—Is Everything Enough?" The title was bannered over the ravishing photo of us posing in our tented living room.

The idea for the story came from the magazine's editor in chief, Clay Felker. Clay was traveling home from Europe when he saw a small photo of Egon and me at a charity ball in Texas in the newsmaker section of *Newsweek*. The ball had been designed by Cecil Beaton and dignitaries had been invited from all over the globe. Egon and I looked particularly glamorous. The young princess was wearing a beautiful, practically topless Roberto Capucci gown and the young prince was breathtakingly handsome in a perfectly cut tuxedo.

Clay, who was the creator of the weekly, decided to assign a pictorial cover story about this young, intriguing couple. A serious feminist writer, Linda Bird Francke, and a highly qualified photographer, Jill Krementz, were assigned the story. There were photos of Egon in the subway, me at the hairdresser, the babies in their nursery, the two of us walking the streets and at an art gallery with Egon's parents. The photos looked very good and the quotes were unusually candid and titillating. Egon teased about having an open bisexual relationship and I compared sex in a marriage to a left hand touching a right one. It sounded so blasé and cynical but we were very young, acting cool at all cost, and, ultimately, very naïve with the press.

The result was shocking and it destroyed our marriage. Reading the magazine and seeing our lives exposed under a magnifying glass, I realized that that couple was not who I was. I didn't want to be a European Park Avenue princess with a pretend decadent life. That woman was definitely not the woman I wanted to be. I had to leave the couple in order to be me. Egon moved out soon after that piece in *New York* magazine, but our friendship and shared family lasted forever.

Egon and I had an easier, deeper, more sincere and respectful relationship after we parted. Of course he was sad and resentful at first, but the breakup was absolutely the only right thing to do, so eventually he accepted it. Parting ways does not mean erasing entirely someone from your life. The relationship can evolve, and be nurtured, but in a different way. Not an easy task, but as anything meaningful, well worth it.

I didn't have to work at being nice to Egon. He was my first true love, the man I married, the one who gave me my children. I never judged him and always loved him; I just could not endorse us as a couple. We remained extremely close for the rest of his life. He was family. When Barry came into my life, we often traveled together with Egon and the children, and we always spent Christmas all together.

I was with Egon in Rome when he died of cirrhosis of the liver in June 2004, two weeks before his fifty-eighth birthday. He had had hepatitis C for a while. He had led a life of excess until his health finally failed him. He had been too ill to come to Cloudwalk and cold Connecticut for Christmas the previous December, so we went to him in Florida and celebrated the holiday with the children and grandchildren in a hotel suite in Miami. As usual, Barry was with us, as was Egon's second wife, Lynn Marshall. My mother was no longer with us, and between missing her and seeing Egon so weak, our reunion that year felt a bit sad. Nonetheless, we were still together, a loving and extended family.

Egon was back in Rome when he was first hospitalized. He was not the type to ever complain, but he started calling more and more frequently to express his worries. Should he, could he have a liver transplant? The children alternated in going to visit him. With Alex he went to a thermal spa hotel in Abano, where his mother, Clara, was already staying with her husband. Then Tatiana went to spend weeks with him at his home in Rome. With his brother, Sebastian, Egon attended his uncle Umberto's funeral. It was his last outing—he had to be rushed back into the hospital again.

Tatiana got to Rome first. Alex and I arrived on the morning of June 10, 2004. It was very hot. We bought fruits in the street and brought them to him. Egon took me aside and asked me to talk to the doctors. He was worried that they were not telling him the truth. I promised I would. We stayed in his room until dusk, talking and laughing a lot. His vision was blurred, but in his unique way of beautifying everything, he referred to the spots he was seeing as intricate embroideries on the wall. He insisted on telling us what restaurant we should go to for dinner, but we didn't want to go to a noisy restaurant. Instead, we hurried back to our tiny connecting rooms at the Hotel Hassler and ordered room service. The three of us wanted to be as close together as we could. We were very worried.

As Egon had asked, I spoke to the doctor and the news was not good. His lungs were filling with fluid, his heart was weak, and his kidneys were failing. I did not discuss it with the children. There was nothing to say. We all knew.

Egon called the next morning as we were having breakfast. He sounded weak and a little breathless. "You'd better come soon," he said, then added, "I hope you can stay a few days. You will have a lot to take care of."

We raced to the hospital, where we found his room filled with emergency staff and machines. Egon seemed agitated and in pain, and we were asked to leave the room. As I walked the corridor feeling helpless, I found myself looking toward the sky, begging, "Stop the suffering." Soon enough we were allowed in again. He had a small oxygen mask on his mouth and nose and was breathing heavily. Alex sat on a chair, sobbing. Tatiana was caressing Egon's head and I was holding his hand when the breathing stopped. He fell silent, empty and at peace. Gently, I closed his eyes. It felt natural, an act of love, of trust, of remembrance for all we had been to each other. I felt honored and privileged to be there.

My first instinct was to protect the children. I felt like a lioness and commanded them out of the room as the nurses came in and, after confirming the death, went about gathering his belongings, covering the body, and rushing him out of the room on a gurney. I followed it down the long corridors, and found myself in no time at all in a room with a man handing me something that looked like a menu. It had photos and prices. "I need your help," I heard myself pleading to the children as they joined me in what I realized was the morgue. "We have to choose the coffin."

At first it was all about arrangements. Egon's godmother and aunt Maria Sole appeared, and together we decided on the mass the next day at Egon's favorite church, the Chiesa degli Artisti on Piazza del Popolo. I asked a friend of the family, Father Pierre Riches, to lead the funeral mass. Maria Sole's daughter, Tiziana, put the announcements in the papers. Egon wanted to be buried in Strobl, Austria, with his father and ancestors. We needed to get the papers from the embassy. Susanna Agnelli, another of Egon's aunts, had been Italy's secretary of state, so her office handled that, and Sebastian, Egon's brother, made the preparations for the funeral in Austria for Monday. It was Friday. All went so fast. Egon was right. There were many things that had to be organized.

The whole family and hundreds of friends rushed to Rome for the funeral. Tatiana and I had chosen the flowers, white lilies, his favorites, and the church service was beautiful—except for the absence of music. I had simply forgotten to arrange for any music. I did, however, arrange a drink at Egon's apartment for his friends after the service, committing apparently a major mistake by bringing the body back home after church. At sunset, a fleet of three cars with handsome, elegant drivers drove Egon to Austria.

Egon's burial was scheduled for Monday. We flew to Salzburg on Barry's plane. Ira, Egon's sister, and her son Hubertus were with us. When we got to Strobl, Egon's coffin was waiting in the library of Hubertushof, the family house on the Wolfgangsee near Salzburg. It is a huge old hunting lodge, which has been passed down from male to male in the Furstenberg line and now belongs to Alexandre. There were flowers everywhere. There, I finally had time to sit by Egon and properly say good-bye.

We had known each other since we were eighteen. We had grown up together, played together, pretended we were adults together, became parents together. Since we had met, our relationship had evolved and changed but we never stopped loving each other. Now he was gone.

I went for a walk alone in the garden, came back, sat at the desk in the library, and wrote him a letter. I had picked a very light paper so I could fold it many times into a small square and I put it on my heart under my bodysuit. Family and friends arrived, drinks and light food were served. At twelve o'clock Egon's casket was put on a carriage pulled by horses. A band accompanied us as we walked slowly from the house to the little church in the center of the village. The sun was shining on the lake.

The service was moving, with music this time, organs. Tatiana read a beautiful speech she had written, so beautiful I had it printed later as a remembrance. Then everyone walked behind the casket to the little churchyard where Egon joined his ancestors in the family graveyard. His burial marked the end of a long tradition. He was the last Furstenberg to be buried there because there is no more room in the vault. I took the letter that was still on my heart and tossed it on the casket when my turn came to throw the dirt. Egon had always loved and kept my letters to him; this one would be with him forever.

For all that it had been my idea to separate from Egon those many years before, I had felt unsettled as most women do when a meaningful relationship ends. I was only twenty-six. Jas Gawronski was in his midthirties, an Italian newsman of Polish origins who reported from New York every night on Italian television. He was very handsome, and the best friend of Egon's uncle Gianni Agnelli. My friendship and love affair with Jas gave me the assurance I craved after the separation from Egon. Our affair was secret at first. One summer, when the children were with their grandmothers, he took me to the little island of Ponza where he had a house. Every day at sunset we used to walk to the top of the mountain and along the whole island to the lighthouse. That is where I discovered the joy of hiking, and to this day, when we sail to Ponza, I always take Barry and the whole family on that same gorgeous hike.

It was Jas who was with me the first night I spent at Cloudwalk, New Year's Eve 1973, when we cooked lamb chops and drank champagne to celebrate the New Year, my new house, and a new life. It was Jas who started to prune the pine trees around the house and it was with him that I went on my first long walk there. Jas was well educated and very kind. He was married but lived apart from his wife. He did not want to commit; nor did I, really. It was a healing period, pleasant and light. My children at home and my dresses at work occupied most of my time. Jas was my personal, private garden even though he and the children did get along fine.

At work I could smell the growing success. The wrap dress was born and selling very well. I was traveling all around America and had become a household name. At home in New York, I lived with my children and my mother. I would dine with them and go out after they went to bed. I felt free and empowered; it wasn't easy managing it all and I was often under huge stress, but it was my choice and well worth it. I felt light traveling with a tiny bag full of jersey dresses and perched on my high heels. It was my turn to feel free and experiment. On a business trip to Los Angeles, I flirted with Warren Beatty and Ryan O'Neal on the same weekend. I was truly living my fantasy of having a man's life in a woman's body. Life was fun if you were young, pretty, and successful in the seventies.

And then I met Barry Diller.

I was twenty-eight when Barry exploded into my life and into our family. I had no idea that this mysterious, successful thirty-three-year-old studio head would become so important to me and my children. We were both young tycoons then: he, the very young chairman of Paramount Pictures; I, the young runaway fashion success. I had read about Barry but I had no inkling of the passion that would overtake us both after we met at a party I gave in my apartment in New York for the powerhouse Hollywood agent Sue Mengers. I remember him coming to my crowded apartment, I remember Sue introducing us, I remember his deep, authoritative voice, and I remember thinking he could be an interesting friend to have. He did not stay long but called me the next morning. He asked me out to dinner that night but when he came to pick me up, I surprised him with a dinner

I'd prepared at home. We ate, sat around briefly. We were both nervous. He left quickly.

I went to Paris the next day. He called me every day, his voice was seductive and, after a few days, he abruptly said, "Why don't you come to Los Angeles for the weekend?" Why not, I thought, intrigued and excited by his commanding tone. Adventure was calling. The flight from Paris to Los Angeles stopped in Montreal. I remember looking for a phone booth to call Jas. I told him I was flying to LA to visit someone I had just met. Looking back, I see how cruel I was, but my total need for honesty just made me do it and I felt freer once I had.

I was so excited to get to Los Angeles I don't think I needed an airplane to fly. Once over Arizona, I disappeared into the bathroom and stayed there until we were about to land. I did my hair, my makeup, changed my clothes, and arrived fresh and looking sassy in a skinny little pin-striped pantsuit with very high platform boots. Barry was at the gate. He had arranged a car for my luggage and I joined him in the yellow E-type Jaguar that he drove. It was a very glamorous welcome; I was in Hollywood and it felt like a movie. He offered me the choice of stopping for drinks at the home of his friend, the legendary producer Ray Stark, or going home. We went home.

That home turned out to be a beautiful hideaway, a California Mediterranean-style house at the end of a long driveway in Coldwater Canyon. An English butler showed me the guestroom where a colorful bouquet of flowers welcomed me. I did not need to freshen up; I was superfresh. I assume we had dinner. I don't remember. What I do remember was cuddling close to him on the living room sofa. Just as abruptly as he had commanded me to come to LA, he said, "Let's go to bed." We were both very nervous, lying frozen in his bed under the blanket. We were actually shaking. We each took a Valium and went to sleep.

The next day he went to work and I went exploring the house. What a mysterious man he was. I knew nothing of his life and I was so curious. The drawers were empty, and the books on the bookshelves did not reveal much either. What I did not know and soon found out is that he had just moved into the house and all of the furniture belonged to Paramount's props department. He came home at midday, we had lunch and hung around the pool. Sexual tension was rising. When we finally succumbed, it was major passion and from the first moment our bodies met he surrendered to me in a way that no one had ever done before. He had certainly never opened himself like that before either, he confessed to me later. Something very special and major had happened and we loved each other passionately from that moment on.

His friends were incredulous. No one had known him with a woman before. That made me feel that I was the most special woman in the world.

Barry was in my life forever after. He was to love me unconditionally, guessing my desires and needs and always impressing me with his unquestioning trust. When I went back to New York after this extraordinary weekend, our lives had changed completely. Barry divided his work and his time between LA and New York, where he lived at the Hampshire House on Central Park South. I would visit him there and he would come to me on Park Avenue. I remember the first time he came to Cloudwalk. The children had gone up the night before with the babysitter and I was to join them with Barry on Saturday. He was terribly anxious about meeting the children. He kept delaying the departure, insisting we first visit his tailor, where he ordered some suits. He kept telling me over and over that he didn't know any children. Finally, in the early afternoon, we arrived.

The minute he got there, he became totally at ease, sinking into the coziest chair by the phone in the living room, where he still sits today. Alexandre and Tatiana were as cool as they always were meeting my friends and his nervousness disappeared instantly. I remember him telling me that left alone with him in the room, four-year-old Tatiana smiled at him, and trying to figure him out, asked, "Who are your friends?" Neither of us remembers his answer but we will never forget her question.

From that moment on, he cherished weekends with us in Connecticut, as we still do decades later. One afternoon, as we were driving back to New York, we saw an old couple crossing Lexington Avenue. As Barry slowed the car down to let the couple, holding on to each other, cross the street, we both had the same thought and the same wish: One day we would be that old couple helping each other to cross the street. We both remember that image vividly although he believes it was Madison Avenue and I am sure it was Lexington.

Barry landed in our family life with a wonderful "everything is possible" attitude.

For Mother's Day, 1976, Barry bought me a tiny little speedboat so the kids could learn to water-ski on Lake Candlewood near Cloudwalk. We had a festive Fourth of July party that year. Mike Nichols came with Candice Bergen, Louis Malle came alone (they were to marry a few years later), director Miloš Forman and writer Jerzy Kosinski were there, and my closest neighbor, socialite Slim Keith, brought her houseguest, the old 1930s and '40s movie actress Claudette Colbert. "Oh, I'd love to go on your yacht," Claudette said to Barry when we told her we had spent the day on our boat. We all had a good laugh over the fact that she had imagined our small speedboat was a yacht. But Claudette must have been clairvoyant, because Barry's taste for boats never went away. The boats just got bigger and bigger.

Barry spoiled us all. He brought the children paraphernalia from his show *Happy Days*, and took us to the Dominican Republic and Disneyland. His house in Los Angeles was a favorite with its pool and his collies, Arrow and Ranger, and he invited the children to the Paramount set where they were shooting *Bad News Bears*. On New Year's Eve, for my twenty-ninth birthday, he took me to a party at Woody Allen's where he gave me twenty-nine loose diamonds in a Band-Aid box.

In March 1976 I was on the cover of *Newsweek*. The same Linda Bird Francke who had done the *New York* magazine article that had ended my marriage with Egon wrote a wonderful seven-page article on my business success. Barry was very proud. That Monday he had a photographer take photos of the magazine on all the newsstands in all the different neighborhoods of New York and made an album for me. I teased him that he left out all the foreign newsstands; my cover ran on every continent. Here we were, two young tycoons, twenty-nine and thirty-four, living a fast life on top of the world!

On the drive to Cloudwalk we often stopped at theaters along the way to study people's reactions at his sneak previews. The first preview we went to was *Won Ton Ton: The Dog Who Saved Hollywood*. Not a big hit. Thankfully, after that, Barry had many blockbusters, such as *Marathon Man, Saturday Night Fever, Grease,* and *Urban Cowboy*. I also remember how anxious he was on Sunday mornings tallying the movie numbers that were called in by his VPs of sales. The ashtray beside our bed would fill quickly as the numbers came in from around the country.

The summer of '77 we decided to take the children on a cross-country drive. We flew to Denver and started out in a rented RV with Barry at the wheel. We were hardly out of the airport and there he was, on the side of the highway, changing a flat tire. We spent four days or so in that camper, which we had named Fantasy 1. We drove from Pike's Peak to Durango in Colorado and visited Monument

Valley on our long way to Lake Powell in Utah, where we'd rented a houseboat that we named *Fantasy 2*. I was in charge of the food, Barry and Alex were in charge of getting us to the right places, and Tatiana was in charge of making the beds, but after two nights in the RV, we opted to sleep in motels along the way instead.

The houseboat had its own challenges. Barry was stressed because he was afraid that the boat would slip its mooring and go by itself over the dam and down the waterfall, so he stayed wide awake all night. As soon as I heard about the dam, I started having a fit because I thought the dam had something to do with nuclear power. I drove Barry crazy about the nuclear fears I was having while Alexandre and Tatiana amused themselves by killing flies, hundreds of which were swarming in the boat. Lake Powell is beautiful, though, and we managed to have lots of fun during the day.

The last leg of the trip was rafting down the Colorado River, but Barry gave up—driving the RV and the houseboat had worn him out—so he left and took shelter in a hotel in Las Vegas while Tatiana, Alexandre, and I ended up going down the river alone with the two boatmen, brothers, and camping out on the shore. We had a wonderful time on the river all day and sleeping under the stars at night, as I expect the boatmen did, too, with the large supply of booze they had taken along. At the end of the rafting trip, Barry picked us up by helicopter at the Grand Canyon and we all flew home exhausted, dirty, and happy.

At the end of 1977, for my thirtieth birthday, I bought myself a beautiful apartment on the twelfth floor of 1060 Fifth Avenue. It was a very large apartment that had belonged to Rodman Rockefeller and had an amazing view over the reservoir of Central Park, where every night we could watch the most extraordinary sunset. My good friend Oscar de la Renta's first wife, Françoise, helped me to decorate it in a style that was both lavish and somewhat bohemian. Huge comfortable velvet sofas, upholstered silk fuchsia walls, leopard carpet, and rose print walls for the master bedroom. Barry moved in with us and I built him his own bathroom and dressing room off our bedroom. He was in LA half the time but we all lived very happily together when he came to New York. We gave huge fun parties to celebrate the movies he produced. The children loved Barry and he loved them in return, though like any reasonable person, he cursed at them when they were naughty. Egon appreciated Barry's involvement and used to joke that the children had "two fathers."

Barry and I went out a lot when he was in New York, and I would go out alone when he was not there. Sometimes I flirted with other men or boys. It was that time in New York; we were very free. Barry did not ask questions, nor did I for that matter. Our relationship was above that. We loved being together and we loved being apart.

I had a little fling with Richard Gere, who had just finished *American Gigolo.* Hard to resist. His agent, Ed Limato, was upset with him and told him that seeing me was not a good move for his career as Paramount distributed the film. Barry never said anything but I know he was not happy. Barry was always cool, above anything and anyone. He knew it would pass.

Studio 54 had opened, and was the final stop for any evening in New York. Sometimes, when Barry was in LA, late at night I would put on my cowboy boots, take my car, park in the garage, walk into 54, meet my friends, have a drink, and dance. What I loved best was going in alone, the long entrance, the disco music. I felt like a cowboy walking into a saloon. But the idea of being able to go to 54 alone is what thrilled me the most: again, a man's life in a woman's body! It was fun. We all felt very free as we did not know yet about AIDS. I never stayed too late though. I had my children and my mother at home and had to wake up early to go to work.

I kept going back and forth to the factories in Italy and would sometimes stop in Paris on the way, to shop and act like a rich American tourist. I remember having tea in the lobby of the Plaza Athénée with my friend, the tall, flamboyant André Leon Talley, who was the *Women's Wear Daily* Paris correspondent at the time. I used to force him to pretend he was an African king.

I had become the woman I wanted to be and I absolutely loved my life. I had two beautiful, healthy children; a wildly successful fashion business; a lot of fun and a wonderful man with whom I shared so much. In 1980, Barry rented a sailboat called *Julie Mother* and he and I sailed the Caribbean. I was reading a fascinating book *The Third Wave* by the futurist writer Alvin Toffler. The book predicted that soon we would communicate through computers, that we would have ways to connect to information and in turn send that information around the world. It sounded wild, like science fiction. I was amazed, underlining paragraphs and taking a lot of notes. I remember my fountain pen had turquoise ink, the color of the sea, on which we were sailing . . . I had a feeling the world would change. It did.

The night we came back, I got the call from Hans Muller. My mother was in bad shape. He needed me to come to Switzerland immediately. I jumped on a plane. After spending a few very difficult weeks in the mental ward of the hospital taking care of my mother and watching her fight her demons, I returned to New York, but things had changed. I felt out of place in my own gilded, easy life. Barry was as loving as ever, but I felt off balance. To see my mother so bad, to relive with her the horrors of her past, took a toll on me. I had to escape the excess of my fast-moving life. I took the children and went as far away as I could: the island of Bali.

"Do your work, then step back. The only path to serenity," wrote the Chinese philosopher Lao Tzu in the sixth century BC. I took that big step back in the summer of 1980 as I walked five miles along a beautiful, peaceful Balinese beach and watched the sun come up on my first day there. New York, Barry, Richard, success—I had run away from it all. That morning, at five a.m., I chanced upon Paulo, a handsome bearded Brazilian with long, curly hair who lived in a bamboo house on the beach and hadn't worn shoes in ten years. I felt so far away and my life took yet another turn. Paulo smelled delicious, a mixture of the frangipani flowers that decorated his house and cloves from the Gudam Garang cigarettes he smoked. He collected and sold textiles, spoke Bahasa Indonesia, and took me and the children to discover all the temples and mysteries of the island. At first it was a vacation affair, a way to forget the terrible weeks of my mother's illness . . . another escape. In retrospect, it should have stayed that way, but it didn't.

I was completely and absolutely infatuated with everything in Bali, including Paulo. I did not think of or wish for a future with him, but I was captivated by the adventure of the unknown. When I returned to New York, there was Barry, looking at me lovingly, searching into my eyes and my heart, being sad. He knew something had changed. I felt terrible, but my rush of emotions was overruling my reason.

My children were not happy with me when Barry moved out and Paulo joined us in New York. Nor was my mother. What was I doing? Was I really in love with that "jungle man"? Was I going to give up

Barry's unconditional love? Everyone was incredulous. I was defiant. More than being in love with Paulo, I was in love with the disruption that love can cause.

Paulo made his official appearance on the New York scene at a dinner I gave in my Fifth Avenue apartment for Diana Vreeland and her book *Allure*. He appeared barefoot, wearing a silk shirt over an ikat sarong from the island of Kupang. Eyebrows were raised, but I didn't care. In fact, I enjoyed it. I was on a mission to be provocative, and craved the adventure of it all.

Paulo was also a constant reminder of Bali, that magical island which had so inspired me with its beauty, its fabrics, and its colors. I created a whole makeup line called Sunset Goddess. I was living the fantasy of being a goddess myself and dedicated a perfume, Volcan d'Amour (Volcano of Love), to my new man. Cloudwalk was soon filled with Indonesian textiles and artifacts and I planted colorful ceremonial flags along the river that are there to this day.

Change followed change when I took the children out of school in New York, moving them permanently to Cloudwalk. I felt a sense of danger in the city. John Lennon had been killed by a deranged fan at the doorway of his building in December 1980, and I was haunted by the kidnapping of Calvin Klein's eleven-year-old daughter, Marci, for ransom. Thankfully she had been released unharmed, but my anxiety persisted. Alexandre and Tatiana were eleven and ten, too old to be taken to school and young enough to be swayed by the temptations of city life and the pseudosophistication of some of their city friends. I wanted them to connect with nature, to do without the constant activities in New York, and develop their own resources and imaginations. With some amazement, I realized there had been value to my periods of childhood boredom in Belgium.

I also made the move because of me. I was less interested in being a tycooness with a fast life than I was in being a more present mother and a more devoted partner to a man. It was a phase, but it was real. I went to New York on Tuesday mornings and was back at Cloudwalk on Thursday nights. Paulo spent his days building a new barn and the children went to Rumsey Hall, a nearby private school.

My makeover extended to my clothes. I gave up wearing my own dresses, which were then being designed by licensees anyway, and wore only sarongs, then replaced my sexy high heels with sandals in the summer and boots in the winter. I wore exotic jewelry and let my hair go very curly, often with a fresh flower in it. Paulo and I traveled back to Bali and his bamboo house on the beach whenever we could. Often the children came along.

Looking back, I smile at the ways I tailored my personality to merge with those of different men at different times in my life. I think most women consciously change their stripes or at least modify them in their relationships with men, especially during the delicious period of seduction. They become instant football lovers or sailing enthusiasts or political junkies, then taper back to their own personalities when the relationship is either cemented or over. No one I know, however, went to the lengths I did.

My relationship with Paulo lasted four years, as did my wardrobe of sarongs. "Why don't you wear real clothes?" my mother kept asking. But even she couldn't envision my next metamorphosis when I left Paulo to become the muse to a writer in Paris.

The summer of 1984, after I sold my cosmetics business to the English pharmaceutical company Beecham, I chartered a sailboat to sail around the Greek islands. The children were young teenagers, their relationship with Paulo was not good, and the mood on board was

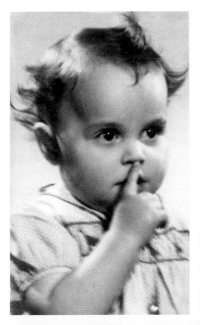

As a toddler,
curious already.

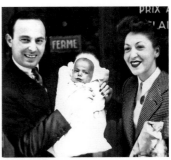

As a baby with
my parents.

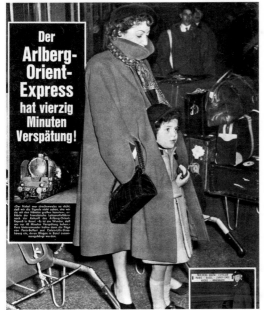

My mother and
I waiting for the
Orient Express,
the first time I
had my photo
in a magazine.

Unless otherwise noted, all photographs courtesy of the author.

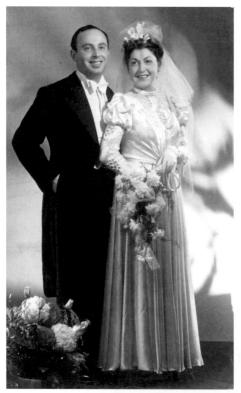

My parents on
their wedding day,
November 29, 1945.

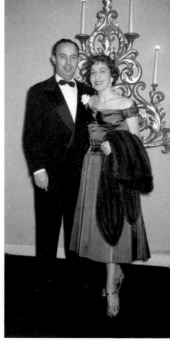

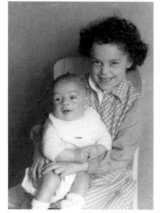

With my
baby brother,
Philippe, in
1953.

My parents going to
a party, 1958.

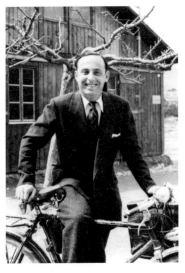

My young father on his bicycle.

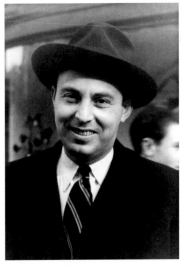

My father, Leon.

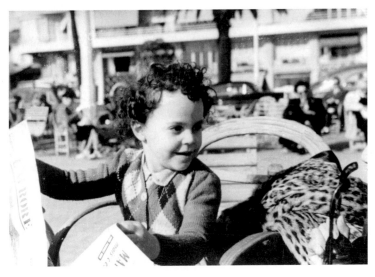

Age three, pretending to read the newspaper.

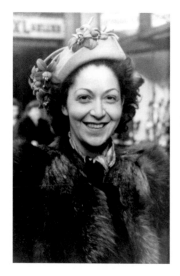

My mother, Lily.

One of the two notes tossed
by my mother en route to the
prison camp in Malines.

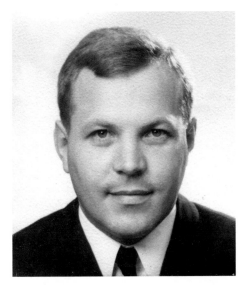

Hans Muller, my mother's longtime companion.

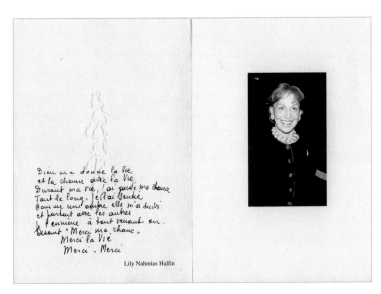

Dieu m'a donné la Vie.
et la chance avec la Vie.
Durant ma Vie, j'ai gardé ma chance
Tout le long, Je l'ai gardée
Comme une amie elle m'a suivi
et partant avec les autres
Je l'emmène à tout venant en.
Disant "Merci ma chance,,
Merci la Vie
Merci - Merci

Lily Nahmias Halfin

My mother's remembrance card featuring a note she wrote to herself.

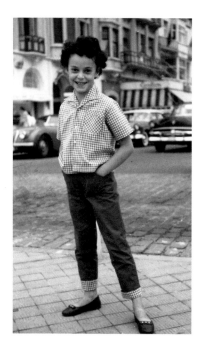

Age nine, in the Belgian resort of Knokke le Zoute.

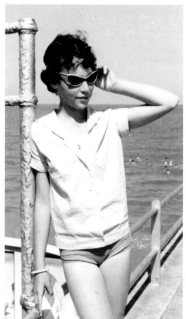

As a preteen on vacation at the North Sea.

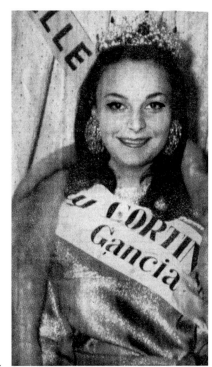

Lady Cortina, my first and only beauty contest, 1967.

At age fifteen, flying solo.

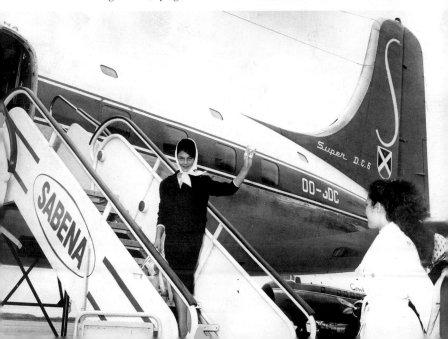

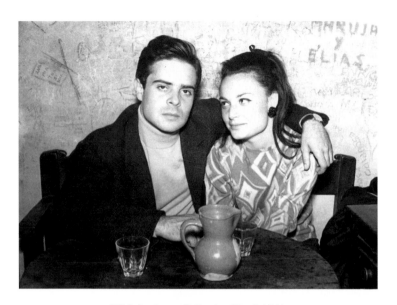

With Lucio, my Italian boyfriend, 1966.

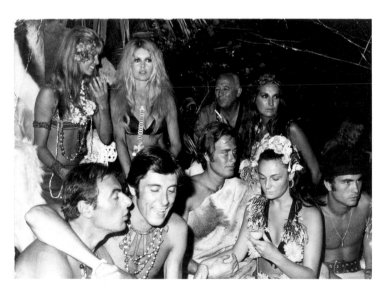

At a pirate-themed party at Brigitte Bardot's in St. Tropez.

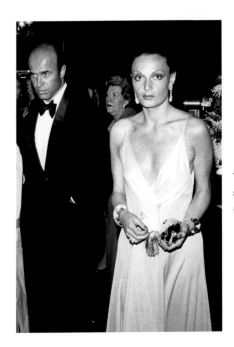

With Jas Gawronski
at a party in 1975.
(Ron Galella, Getty image)

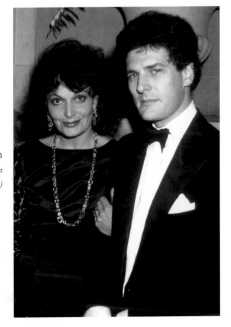

With Alain Elkann in
New York, 1986. *(Ron
Galella, Getty image)*

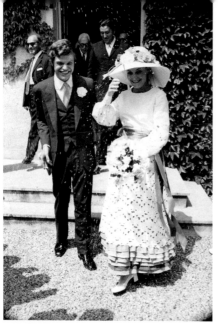

On my wedding day with Prince Eduard Egon von und zu Fürstenberg in Montfort-l'Amaury, near Paris, on July 16, 1969.
(Berry Berenson Perkins)

Egon and I in our Park Avenue apartment in the early 70s.
(Horst, Condé Nast, Corbis Image)

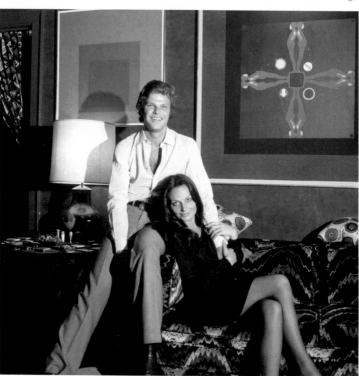

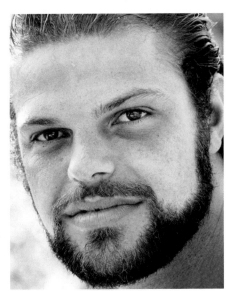

Egon in 1972.

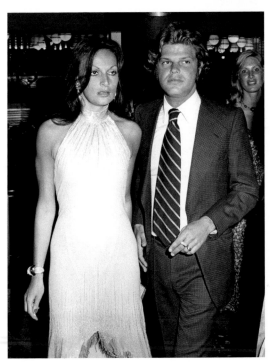

Egon and I at a
party in New York
1970. *(Ron Galella,
Getty image)*

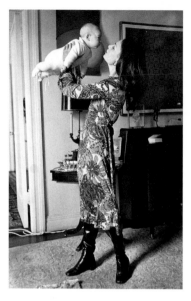

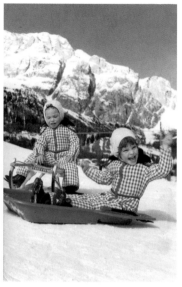

With my baby son, Alexandre, 1970.

Alexandre and Tatiana during winter vacation in Cortina d'Ampezzo.

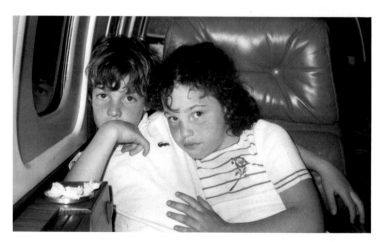

Alexandre and Tatiana on our way to vacation, 1977.

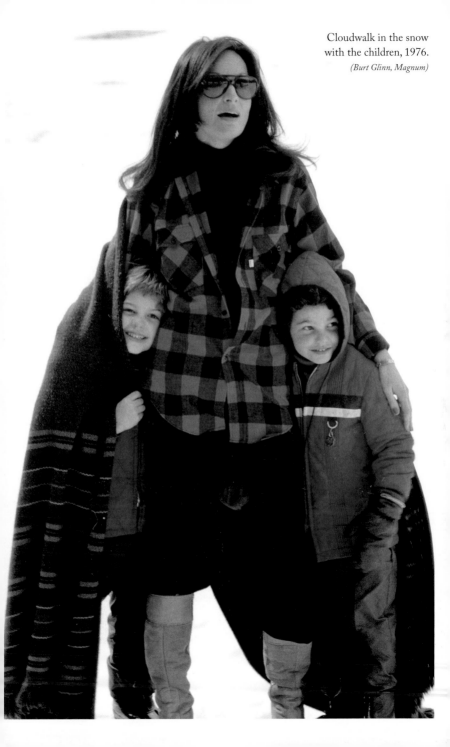

Cloudwalk in the snow
with the children, 1976.
(Burt Glinn, Magnum)

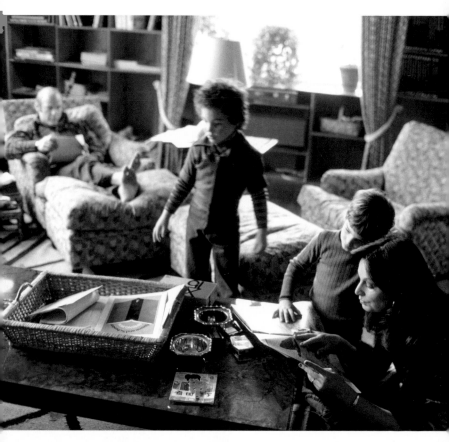

Cloudwalk living room in 1976 with Barry and the children. *(Burt Glinn, Magnum)*

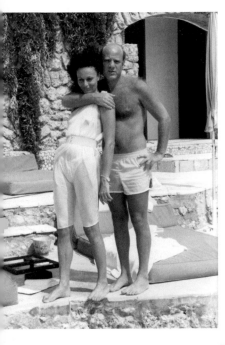

With Barry in
Santo Domingo,
1977.

At the premiere of the
movie *Grease*, 1978.

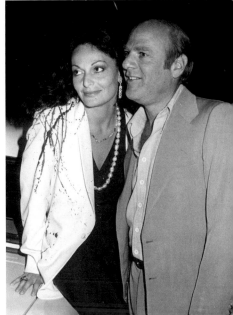

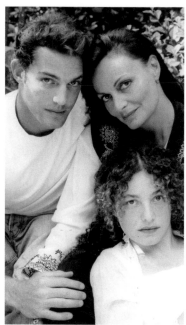

With the grown-up children, 1992. *(Wayne Maser, courtesy of the artist)*

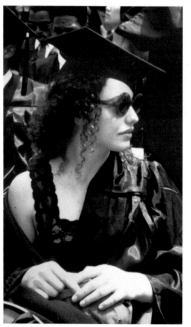

Tatiana graduates from Brown University at nineteen!

heavy and unpleasant. My close Brazilian friend Hugo Jereissati, who had first led me to discover Bali, was with us. I remember telling Hugo while we were sunbathing, "My life is going to change again." It did.

Wool skirts. Buttoned-up sweaters. Flat shoes. They would dominate my wardrobe for the next five years. Alain Elkann, an Italian novelist and journalist, didn't like the sexy clothes I had just started designing, so, yet again, I changed my stripes for love. My new image startled me every time I looked in the mirror.

I'd met Alain in New York at a fourteenth-birthday party Bianca Jagger was giving for her daughter, my goddaughter Jade. Tatiana and Alex were both home from boarding school, she from England and he from Massachusetts, and we were all in New York that weekend.

Alain was very attractive and we knew a lot of people in common as he had been married to Margherita Agnelli, Egon's first cousin. "Come with me to Paris," Alain said soon after we met. I didn't hesitate. The children were away at school and I couldn't bear another day in New York. Just as I had found Paulo during my introspection after my mother's collapse, I found Alain in 1984 during my disenchantment with New York. Life in New York had become all about money—*Dynasty* and *Dallas* were the hits on television—and after four years cloistered at Cloudwalk with Paulo, Paris intellectual life was very appealing to me. My work wasn't really interesting anymore. Though I was working on starting a new business, my heart wasn't really in it.

What was in my heart was Alain. And Paris. Paulo was very angry and moved to his native Brazil; I moved to a beautiful apartment I rented on rue de Seine between a courtyard and a garden. My friend François Catroux, an interior decorator, helped me to set up a chic and bohemian interior filled with Empire furniture and the pre-Raphaelite paintings from my recently sold Fifth Avenue apartment.

Alain and I entertained a lot: writers, artists, and designers, even though fashion was no longer my priority. Alain had a day job at Mondadori, the publishing house, and wrote novels after work. My all-time favorite writer, Alberto Moravia, stayed with us for weeks at a time. He would write in the morning, and in the afternoons he and I would go to museums, movies, or to Café de Flore for hot chocolate. I could not believe we had become such close friends.

In my new Parisian life I rediscovered my first love, literature, and was living yet another fantasy—having a literary salon and founding a small publishing house, Salvy, where we published in French the great writers Vita Sackville-West, Gregor von Rezzori, and Bret Easton Ellis, among others.

Alain and I also had a lively, loving family life during holidays. He had three children with Margherita Agnelli: John ("Jaki"), Lapo, and Ginevra. Maybe because they were related to my own children, we immediately became a family. We only had the five children on vacations and occasional weekends, but took full advantage of the time. We skied together in Gstaad, swam in Capri where Alain and I rented a small apartment, and sailed up the Nile to discover ancient Egypt. The rest of the time I was with Alain, the perfect writer's muse, listening to his writings and following his many moods. I ran a perfect intellectual stylish home, with abundant food and fresh flowers at all times. I had long known that writers may live the bohemian life, but they love luxury. I set up a small office on the attic floor and talked to my very reduced New York office daily.

For all that I loved my life in Paris, being with Alain was sometimes difficult. Though I shared his life and interests entirely, he did not share mine. In 1986, I was one of eighty-seven immigrants chosen to receive a Mayor's Liberty Award for my contribution to the city of New York and the United States. I was very proud and wanted to go to New York for the ceremony and receive my award from Mayor Ed Koch, but Alain did not want me to go, so I didn't. My mother went for me.

Looking back, I realize how many things I let go for my relationship with Alain. He wanted me to give up my personality and my success and I actually did it with enthusiasm. No one had ever asked me that before. I traded my passion for independence to be "the woman of." My children were astonished. "Mommy has zero personality," they used to say, and I smiled. I knew deep down it wasn't really true, but I was seduced by the role I was embracing of the devoted artist's woman.

All probably would have continued except I came to realize that Alain was having an affair with my good friend Loulou de la Falaise, muse of Yves Saint Laurent. Loulou was all the things I had given up: glamour, work, success. I was shocked, very sad, and upset at first, but I grew to understand on some level that it was, at least partially, my fault. By altering my personality, I had lost what had attracted Alain to me in the first place. I had become the docile, passive person I thought he wanted only to have him stray toward the same sort of person I had been. I am not one to accept humiliation, however, and instead, I turned the betrayal into a determination to win. By staying cool when I confronted them and exposed the affair, I trusted my calm attitude would diminish the lure of the "forbidden fruit" and eventually destroy it. I was right. The affair soon lost its appeal and ended. Alain and I stayed together a bit more, but I knew it would soon be time to move on.

In retrospect, I would not give up those years in Paris with Alain or the years with Paulo in and out of Bali for anything in the world. No one goes through life with one rigid personality. We are far more complex with various needs and desires that present themselves at different stages of our lives. Because I worked for and achieved financial independence so early in life, I had the unusual luxury of fully living those fantasies, and also having the ability to leave them when the time was right.

Paulo gave me the serenity I needed to heal from my mother's collapse and a refuge from the frenetic pace of my life in New York. Alain gave me my return to Europe and the world of culture and ideas I craved after closeting myself at Cloudwalk. Alain also gave me three wonderful stepchildren whom I love and have stayed close to. Jaki is now the respected John Elkann who runs Fiat motor company and its subsidiaries, Lapo is a very successful designer and a marketing genius, and Ginevra is a princess, mother of three, film producer, and president of Pinacoteca Giovanni e Marella Agnelli. All three are siblings to Alex and Tatiana and we are a family.

I've often asked myself what sort of woman I'd be today if I hadn't experimented with such greatly different lifestyles with Paulo and Alain. Would I have been ready all those years ago to stay with Barry? Part of me wishes I had instead of hurting him and losing the years we could have spent together. But another part of me is glad. I'm probably a better wife and partner to Barry now because of it. I needed to try on different versions of myself to see which one fit me best. And after Alain I still wasn't through.

My personal life was in limbo when I left Paris in 1989 and returned to New York. As usual, Barry was there to listen to me and reassure me, but to some degree we had lost each other and I did not want to hurt him again. I had to find myself first and that was not easy. I divided my time between Cloudwalk, the Carlyle Hotel in New York where I took an apartment, and the Bahamas where I helped my mother to settle into her little white house with blue shutters on the pink sand beach of Harbour Island.

I also renewed old friendships, and had some flirtations, but I really was not happy with myself. As much as I loved Barry's company—we went everywhere together—I still wasn't ready to commit. One of the reasons was that I had started a secret relationship with a handsome, mysterious, talented man, the only man who would, in the end, leave me.

I didn't mean to fall in love with Mark Peploe, nor he, I'm sure, with me. Mark had been a friend for a long time and had written the screenplay for Bernardo Bertolucci's *The Last Emperor* in the guest room when I lived with Alain in Paris. (It won nine Academy Awards in 1988, including Best Adapted Screenplay.) Mark also was "taken"—he lived with a woman I knew and their twelve-year-old daughter in London. It never occurred to me to have an affair with him until he called me one day in New York after I'd returned from Paris—and sparks flew.

It was the stuff of fantasy. Literally. When I was a young girl, I used to write poetry and short stories about love and always thought that stolen moments, the untold, the unasked, the secrecy, defined the most exciting and romantic relationships. And our affair was exactly that. Mark and I had a great relationship; I respected his intellect, he was one of the most handsome men I'd ever met, and he was a great traveling companion. Soon after our affair began he asked me to join him in Sri Lanka where he was scouting sites for *Victory,* a movie he was going to direct. I barely knew where Sri Lanka was, or that it was the new name for Ceylon. I immediately booked a flight.

I will never forget driving around the island of Serendib, the magical island that gave us the word "serendipity," with Mark, discovering the rubber and tea plantations, the reclining Buddha, the house of the author Paul Bowles, and the streets of Colombo. We were so far from everything. I was in awe of this elegant, handsome man who knew so much ... our conversations were endless. They continued in all different landscapes—the streets and cafés of Paris, the trattorias of Rome, the streets of Lisbon, the souks and the harem of Topkapi in Istanbul, the Byzantine caves of Cappadocia, the Sufi mosque of Konya, the Vermillion Cliffs in Utah, and in discovering the artist Mantegna in Mantova. All through these landscapes, we talked and talked about everything. When traveling by car, I would read aloud the traveling adventures of the Polish journalist Ryszard Kapuscinski, or the passions of the Austrian writer Stefan Zweig. Those were our stolen moments, stolen from our everyday lives in anonymous hotels, airports, and rented cars.

Barry knew about Mark and Mark knew about Barry, although I avoided talking much about one to the other. I now realize that Barry was already like my husband and Mark was my secret lover. I could not give up one for the other. I must have been cruel to both, but I did not think I was at the time. Barry was waiting patiently, secure of the outcome. What was really in Mark's mind, I never knew. I loved our "unspoken relationship," and wanted it to go on and on, but it didn't.

I felt great pain when Mark left me for yet another woman, not the mother of his child. I thought he enjoyed the fantasy of our secret relationship as much as I did, but perhaps he'd wanted a more permanent and visible relationship. He never explained, I never asked.

In retrospect, I know that Barry's existence and my feelings for him had everything to do with my reluctance to commit fully to Mark,

Alain, or Paulo. After Mark and I parted, Barry began taking up more and more space in my life, in my bed, and in my heart, and we found a new serenity.

Sailing the oceans, we found a way to design our lives together. Barry had had a love affair with boats ever since I'd taken him with me on *Atlantis,* the elder Stavros Niarchos's sublime yacht, when the children were very small and spending the summer with Egon. That time we'd cruised the Amalfi Coast all the way to Greece. It was a revelation for Barry, the beginning of a dream to one day build his own yacht. We took many wonderful trips after that on chartered boats to the Mediterranean, the Caribbean, the Ionian Coast. I had always loved to travel to adventurous places, he needed his luxury and to be connected to his work. On those sailing trips we could do both . . . go on adventurous inland hikes, visit small villages, and yet come back to our floating comfort and communications at night.

We had always talked about our future over the years and we both knew we would end up together. I loved Barry and knew he was absolutely the only one I could marry, but I fought the notion of marriage itself. People often refer to it as "settling down," and the words are so uninspiring to me. "Settle down" sounds like giving up your spontaneity and independence and that was not what I, or Barry for that matter, were about.

I began to soften when he started talking about marriage out of concern for the children. He wanted to be able to provide for them, he said, and marriage would make it much easier. When Alexandre married Alexandra Miller in 1995 (thus becoming Alex and Alex), Barry gave him a jar of earth as a wedding present to represent a sum of money for the down payment on a house. He was so sincere about caring for my children, I was moved.

My journals in 1999 tracked various family milestones. The birth of Talita, my first grandchild, was, of course, a major milestone. Another was that Tatiana was pregnant. She had wanted a baby so badly that when we went together to visit little Talita, she had gone outside and cried in a phone booth fearing she would never have one. The very next day she met Russell Steinberg, a loving, life-happy comedian. Antonia Steinberg was born one year and twenty-two days after Talita's birth, the exact same length of time between Tatiana and Alexandre. My diary notes another milestone: I finally paid off my mortgage on Cloudwalk. The last entry was not yet a milestone: "Talking marriage with Barry," I wrote.

It didn't happen in 1999. It didn't happen in 2000, but Barry did not give up hope. "Today, for my birthday Barry gave me a pearl ring that belonged to Marie Bonaparte and a card with a wish to marry," I wrote in my journal. Another entry was sad. "Lily not well," I noted, as my mother's health continued to slip away. Alexandre was in Australia, but the rest of the family, including my brother, Philippe, all gathered at her house in Harbour Island for Easter. Remarkably, she managed to hang on and pull together what strength she had left to fly with me to Los Angeles to be there with Tatiana for the birth of baby Antonia. It was during that flight that I told her I was thinking of maybe marrying Barry, to which she gloriously replied: "He deserves you."

How I loved my mother for saying that! She did not say I deserved him, she said he deserved me. In those three words was everything—how she valued me, the person I had become, and how she valued him for deserving me. I will never forget that. Not only had she given me her approval for marrying Barry, she was telling me how proud she was of me. She died a few weeks later.

I needed another approval—Egon's. I called him and said I was considering marrying Barry. "I want your blessing," I said to him. "You have it, but keep my name," he answered, laughing.

A week before Barry's fifty-ninth birthday, as I was looking for a present to give him, I decided to give him myself. "Why don't we get married on your birthday?" I casually said over the phone. "Let me see if I can arrange it," he answered with no hesitation. "Let me see if I can arrange it" is something he'd taken on from the minute we met ... and always delivered. Sure enough, he arranged for us to marry at City Hall a week later.

I called the children, I called my brother in Belgium, and I called my friend, the world-famous portrait photographer Annie Leibovitz, to ask her if she could come and take the photos. Philippe flew into New York with his wife, Greta, and daughters, Kelly and Sarah. Tatiana flew in from Los Angeles with Russell and little eight-month-old Antonia strapped to his chest in a baby carrier. Alexandre and his pregnant wife, Alexandra, and twenty-month-old Talita were already in New York. We all met up the morning of the wedding in my design studio, a carriage house on West Twelfth Street, before going down to City Hall. I hadn't thought about flowers but happened to have met a florist a few nights before who offered to make me a wedding bouquet. I chose lilies of the valley to honor my mother. I made myself a cream jersey dress. I did not feel particularly pretty that day, but I was so happy.

As we left the studio, the DVF girls were screaming good wishes. We were met at City Hall by Annie Leibovitz, who, with great generosity, had answered my call and agreed to act as paparazzi. There were, of course, also real paparazzi, but they were not allowed to come with us into City Hall. We were all laughing, my little family and I. It all felt perfectly natural. Barry had arranged a lunch at some obscure restaurant near City Hall. The restaurant was a bit stiff and gloomy, so we did not stay long, but laughed the whole time, though we all missed my mother.

Long before we decided to marry that day, I had planned a big Aquarius party for that night at the studio on Twelfth Street because my three loves, Barry, Tatiana, and Alex, were all born under the sign of Aquarius. The hundreds of friends who joined us for that Aquarius party were startled and overjoyed to discover that it had turned into a wedding celebration! As a present, Barry gave me twenty-six wedding bands with diamonds . . . "Why twenty-six?" I asked. "For the twenty-six years we were not married," he answered.

It took me a while to accept that we were married. When I drove out to the country the next day I saw that someone had put a sign in my car that said "Just Married." I stopped in the middle of the road and turned it over. There was still that rebelliousness in me, and yet when I got to Cloudwalk I was so happy to see Barry already there waiting for me. It was not until quite recently that I actually started referring to Barry as "my husband," but now I do, and I do it with pride and much love. We so love being together. What we like best is to be quiet and alone. We are definitely soul mates and I am forever thankful to Sue Mengers for introducing me to this glamorous young tycoon thirty-nine years ago and to have seduced him forever.

How can I explain my relationship with Barry? The fullness of it all? It is simply true love. His openness to me, his unconditional acceptance, his deep desire for my happiness and that of the children brings tears to my eyes to think about. Barry has a reputation for being tough, yet he is the gentlest, most loving person I have ever met. We have been in each other's lives for decades, as lovers, as friends, and now as husband and wife. It is true that, as I did with my father, I took his love for granted. It is true that, as I did to my father, I sometimes rejected him. But it is also true, as it was with my father, that I love him totally and am there for him unconditionally. Love is life is love is Barry.

We spend at least three months a year on *Eos*, the dream boat Barry finally built. Named for the Greek goddess of dawn, *Eos* took more than three years to build, three years during which Barry spent at least two hours a day going over every detail, talking to the engineers, talking to the construction people in Germany, involving himself in the outside design, inside decoration, and every detail of everything on board. Launched in 2006, *Eos* is the most wonderfully comfortable yacht you can imagine, with a dream crew that creates extraordinary itineraries and always finds the best places for us to hike, and a young, talented chef, Jane Coxwell, who I encouraged to write a cookbook that all of my friends love.

We asked our friend, the artist Anh Duong, to do a sculpture for the figurehead of the boat and she asked me to pose for it. So, there I am in front of *Eos*, sailing the world, literally. With *Eos*, we've been to the Mediterranean and the Red Sea, to Egypt and Jordan. We've been to Oman, the Maldives and Borneo, Thailand and Vietnam. We've spent weeks in Indonesia and discovered the Pacific islands of Vanuatu, Fiji, and Papua New Guinea. Every morning we take a long swim in a new sea, and every afternoon we hike a new path. We have traveled thousands and thousands of miles this way. And we still keep going, exploring new horizons with our dog, Shannon. I take hundreds of pictures that I download at night on my computer. It is bliss to be on *Eos*, our floating home.

Traveling the world with the children and the grandchildren is our happiest time: holidays on the sea, the Galapagos or Tahiti, or on land on safari in Africa or skiing. Sometimes we only take the grandchildren. We forget they are grandchildren and we think they are our children. Years have passed and yet it feels the same as our first trip to Colorado and Lake Powell.

The most important thing Barry and I have in common is that we are both self-reliant. The presence in each other's lives was never a necessity, and therefore always felt like a huge luxury. Barry's generosity warmed me from the minute I met him and that feeling continues to evolve. He is generous with his heart, with his protection, with everything. "We," to us, is home, cozy and reassuring. Our love is our home. We are slowly becoming the old couple that crossed Lexington Avenue, guarding each other. "We" is also our family: the children aging, the grandchildren growing—Love is life is love is life.

Recently, as Barry was remodeling our house in Beverly Hills, he sent me this note:

"I'm in the plane after meeting at the house with the construction team. The house is going to be uniquely dazzling. We're going to have a slate roof and all glass bronze doors and we made your mezzanine room with full glass skylights, and glass sides—a little tree house garden in the sky.

"Hopefully, we'll add another place to grow old gloriously and glamorously. And in the meantime I'm so proud of what you accomplish every day in building your brand and your legacy . . .

"I love you, my honey."

And I love you, Barry.

3

BEAUTY

I am at a birthday party in Brussels for my best friend, Mireille, who is turning ten. As if it were yesterday, I remember us children around the dining room table at her elegant Avenue Louise apartment. The large, fancy cake is about to appear when we hear the hurried click click of a woman's heels in the hallway. Mireille's mother makes her entrance, dressed smartly in a pin-striped suit, her narrow skirt forcing her to take small steps, her makeup and auburn hair perfectly arranged. She is so glamorous and in charge. "*Joyeux anniversaire, ma chérie*—happy birthday, darling," she says to Mireille, kissing her on both cheeks while adjusting her hair. She blows kisses to all of us. The heart-shaped cake is brought in and she watches Mireille blow out the candles, directs the cake cutting, has a piece herself for good luck, talks briefly to each of us, admires our presents, and then, as we go back to Mireille's room to play, she click clicks back down the hall and out the front door.

I am awed. Though it may have been upsetting to Mireille to have her mother be too busy in her life outside the home to spend but the barest time inside, even for her daughter's birthday party, I am filled with wonderment at this glamorous, confident, engaged woman. I know vaguely that Mireille's mother, Tinou Dutry, is a leading businesswoman in Brussels. What I am totally sure of is that I want to be like her when I grow up. Decades later, I realize that my best friend's mother, a proud pioneer who created Belgium's organization for women entrepreneurs and who had been a resistance fighter during the war, was one of my early inspirations for the woman I wanted to be.

I felt the same admiration watching my mother get dressed to go out, whether at night to a party with my father, or by herself during the day. She took great care in what she wore, and her outfit was often punctuated by a hat. Her hair, her makeup, her perfume . . . she looked at herself in the mirror with a smile of complicity and confidence. She had a great figure and wore very tight skirts and dresses. Her heels clicked, too. Where is she going? I wondered. How does she know how to put herself together so well and always look so chic? I couldn't get enough of it, watching all the shine, the allure, the glamour that was my mother. She, too, was the woman I hoped to be.

I did not like my reflection in my mother's mirror. I saw a square, pale face. Brown eyes. And short brown, very, very, very densely curled hair made even more so by the humidity and incessant rain in Brussels. Almost all the girls in my class, including Mireille, had straight, blond hair, which they could have cut with big straight bangs. Not me. I felt alien. I looked like someone who'd snuck out of the forest. No one else looked like that.

I obsessed over my curly hair, which even my skillful mother couldn't deal with. When I returned from two weeks at a summer camp, she got frustrated spending the longest time untangling my hair. She finally succeeded in pulling it into a neat ponytail, braided it, and asked me for my hair clip. I had lost it at camp. After all her effort she got so irritated that she took a pair of scissors and cut the ponytail off. This did not improve what I saw in the mirror. I was miserable and full of shame.

What I did not know until I was told quite recently was that one boy in my kindergarten class loved me *because* of my hair. He, in fact, so adored my brown curls and my brown eyes that he asked me to marry him—and I evidently accepted! How embarrassing to have forgotten my five-year-old first husband, but I had until a few years ago, when I was invited to Belgium to speak to a group of businesswomen. After my talk, which included my childhood and probably a mention of my frustrations with my loathsome hair, Bea Ercolini, the editor of the Belgian edition of *Elle* magazine, asked me what school I had gone to, what years, et cetera, and then she connected the dots. "I think I live with the man you 'married' in kindergarten," she told me, smiling.

"What is the name of this gentleman?" I asked skeptically. "Didier van Bruyssel," she answered. Suddenly, it all started to come back to me. Some of it, anyway. I didn't remember Didier specifically, but I did remember the sound of his name and how, as a child, I had carefully practiced writing my signature with our combined names, Diane van Bruyssel, over and over. I was astonished that Bea had figured out that I was the little girl her partner had told her about. It showed how much she loved him, how carefully she had listened to his childhood stories. It also showed what an unexpected impact I had had on this five-year-old boy in kindergarten.

The point of all this is not to document my first seduction, but how wrong I was to be sad about not having straight blond hair. While I had been desperate to look the same as the other girls, Didier loved me because I was different. When finally we met after five decades, he told me that he had had no idea that "la petite Diane" with the curly hair had become Diane von Furstenberg, but as a little girl I had such an impact on him that he'd continued to look for Mediterranean-looking women with wavy hair. While I'd thought I was such an odd duck, he personified the familiar idiom "Beauty is in the eye of the beholder."

I wrestled with my curls for years and years, watching the weather and seeing humidity as the enemy, wearing scarves, falls, and straightening my hair with all kinds of tools. I ironed it on an ironing board at times, and had it blown out by hairdressers all over the world, convinced that straight hair was the key to beauty and happiness.

It was not until I was almost thirty that I discovered my curls could be an asset. The realization came about after my friend Ara Gallant, a very talented makeup artist/hair stylist turned photographer, was hired to photograph me for the cover of *Interview* in March 1976. Ara was a creature of the night, so it was no surprise that we shot in a studio well after midnight. Ara knew how to make anyone look sexy. He took scissors and made jagged cuts in the black bodysuit I was wearing. After shooting a few rolls, he started to spray my long and very straight hair with water. I was horrified! "Don't worry," he said. "We already have the cover, but I want to photograph you with wet hair." He shot me as my hair was drying into its true curls. A few days later, when I saw the two options for the cover, there was no question as to which one was better . . . The next day I let my hair dry naturally and it was the first time I wore my curls with pride and enjoyed being me. My "new" look was confirmed at a birthday party at Studio 54 for Mick Jagger's then wife, Bianca, who rode around the stage on a white horse at midnight as we all sang happy birthday. "You look like Hedy

Lamarr," the dashing designer Halston told me, referring to a movie star of the 1930s. I was not sure at the time who Hedy Lamarr was, but I knew it was a compliment. My curly hair had become an asset. I felt confident and free.

That confidence didn't stay with me all the time. My hair became a barometer for my self-esteem, and in the early nineties I started to straighten my hair again. Those were not great years. I was yet again in search of myself and was a bit insecure. As I regained confidence, I let the curls come back. I learned how to master them, how to use them and let them be a part of the true me. I even started to welcome humidity because it adds so much volume to curly hair.

It might seem trivial to give that much importance to hair, but I know all women with curls will identify with this struggle. So will some curly-haired men, I recently discovered. During a vacation last year on the boat of a friend, entertainment mogul David Geffen, I was having a conversation about hair with the women on board when Bruce Springsteen the macho, superhero rock star chimed in. He, too, used to hate his Italian curls when he was fifteen and starting out, he confessed, and so did his teenage band mates, The Castiles. They all wished they could switch their Mediterranean curls for straight bangs like the Beatles. So, at night, they would go secretly to a beauty parlor for black women in Freehold, New Jersey, to have their hair straightened! Bruce said he would also sneak into his mother's bathroom, steal some of her long hair pins, comb his hair all on one side, anchor it with the pins, and sleep on that same side to keep it flattened and straight. However, he never managed to achieve the cherubic, pageboy style of John, Paul, George, and Ringo.

My mother had no patience with my dissatisfaction with my appearance and my obsession with my hair. She dressed me in nice clothes and made sure I was always presentable, but beauty was not a worthwhile subject of conversation. She was much more interested in teaching me literature, history, and most of all, to be independent. Indeed, not considering myself beautiful as a young girl turned out to be a plus. Yes, I envied the blond, straight-haired girls, especially Mireille, who was striking to more than just me and would go on, at age seventeen, to marry Prince Christian von Hanover, twenty-seven years her senior. But being too beautiful as a child, I realized as I grew older, can be a curse. Counting too much on your appearance limits one's growth. Looks are fleeting and cannot be your only asset.

Early on I decided that if I could not be a pretty blonde like the other girls, I would accept being different, develop my own personality, and become popular by being funny and daring. I made lots of friends in boarding school as I did later in Geneva, where I lived with my mother and Hans Muller. I was considered "the fun girl," always ready to go and do anything, and people sought me out for that, including Egon, who arrived in Geneva a year after I did. Looking at pictures of those years, I realize that I did have a slim and agile body, long legs, good skin and was, in fact, quite pretty, but I didn't feel it, so my priority was developing a personality.

Though I believed personality, authenticity, and charm were what made a person attractive, along the way I did have many moments of awkwardness and insecurity. I remember my first visit to the Agnellis' house in Cortina d'Ampezzo over the Christmas holidays when I was turning twenty. The Agnellis were the leading family in Cortina and Egon and his younger brother, Sebastian, were the hottest, most eligible boys in the Alpine town. On my last night there, we went to a party where, to my great surprise, I was voted Lady Cortina. Although elegant enough in a lamé dress in rainbow colors, I remember feeling embarrassed and inadequate as I accepted my beauty award. Clearly it was not for my looks, but because I was Egon's girlfriend. They placed a silly rhinestone tiara on top of the hairpiece that was giving my straightened hair more volume and draped me with a Lady Cortina band. I felt foolish and that was visible in my photo on the front page of the local paper the next morning.

I was better prepared the next year when once again I arrived in Cortina on Egon's arm. By then I had lost some of the baby fat on my face, was a bit more polished, and much more at ease with Egon's Italian aristocratic friends. My transformation did not go unnoticed. Years later, Mimmo, a close friend of Sebastian and the son of Angelo Ferretti, my future mentor, reminded me how I'd gone from looking pudgy and awkward one year to looking beautiful and sexy the next. The pictures of those two holidays prove that confidence and ease can make the same person look quite different.

Egon was my guide and my Pygmalion in his world of beautiful, sophisticated people, all of whom seemed to live magical lives drifting from the Alps in the winter to the South of France in the summer and going to party after party in between.

I will never forget the costume ball he took me to in Venice given by Countess Marina Cicogna during the film festival. That weekend was a crash course in glamour. Marina Cicogna was a very successful producer of Italian cinema at the time, working with directors like Fellini, Pasolini, and Antonioni. There were many movie stars at the party: Liz Taylor and Richard Burton; Jane Fonda and Roger Vadim; Audrey Hepburn and her Italian husband, Andrea Dotti; Catherine Deneuve and David Bailey; the gorgeous model Capucine, who had been in *The Return of the Pink Panther*; and the young actor Helmut Berger with director Lucchino Visconti. I remember meeting

Gualtiero Jacopetti, the director of the very provocative new genre documentary, *Mondo Cane*. Gualtiero was a lot older, but very handsome and seductive. We talked all night and I felt beautiful because he paid me so much attention. I was to find out later that he specialized in courting young girls.

I was barely twenty, and only beginning to feel comfortable in Egon's world. I did not smile as easily as he did and he reprimanded me for appearing cold and detached. Slowly, as I felt more comfortable, I warmed up and began to stand on my own. For that party, the most glamorous, fun party I've ever been to, I dressed like a page boy in black midknee velvet pants and a matching jacket with white satin lapels, inspired by Yves Saint Laurent who had just created the tuxedo for women. Mine was definitely not a Saint Laurent; I don't remember where I found the jacket, but I'd had the pants made to my specifications. I wore black tights and thick-heeled shoes with rhinestones. I felt very stylish.

Egon's cousins, the counts Brandolini, and all their aristocratic friends dressed as hippies, all of that being new and daring in a Venetian palace. We danced all night, ate spaghetti at dawn, and watched the sun come up from the cafés of Piazza San Marco holding our shoes in our hands. The next day, the crowd met at the Lido, under the elegant striped cabanas where the parade of gorgeous women in beach attire spent the day under the critical scrutiny of the powerful doyenne of Venice, the Countess Lily Volpi. Exotic Brazilian star Florinda Bolkan and Yul Brynner's beautiful wife, Doris, were there along with all the other beauties, an endless inventory of what appeared to be effortless elegance and class. I was new to the scene and in awe of so much glamour, style, and allure. I wanted to be one of these stylish women in their thirties and could not wait to get older. I wanted to become one of those women across the room who look so poised and seductive.

I am always asked who the women are whose beauty and style inspired me. My favorite compliment as a young girl was being told that I looked like the French actress Anouk Aimée. Sophisticated, incredibly seductive with a deep sexy voice, always playing with her hair and crossing and uncrossing her legs, she was who I wanted to be. Her most famous movie, *Un homme et une femme* (*A Man and a Woman*) had a big impact on me. Anouk and I later became friends. She and I felt enormous simpatico and I often call her when I go to Paris. She lives in Montmartre with her many dogs and cats, the voice on her answering machine is as sexy as ever, and she has many admirers. Once a femme fatale, always a femme fatale!

The epitome of femme fatale will always be Marlene Dietrich, the most glamorous woman of all time. She had the best legs, an extraordinary voice, and a personal style and elegance as no one else. Her strength, courage, and independence were imposing. I never met her but so wished I had especially after I read her memoir, *Nehmt nur mein Leben* (*Just Take My Life*). She had been very brave during World War II, turning her back on the entreaties of the Nazi government in her native Germany and instead promoting US War Bonds and entertaining the Allied troops on the front lines in Algeria, Italy, France, and England. She laughed, sang, drank, cooked, cared little for convention, and had sexual liaisons with men and women into her seventies. She was a free spirit and an inspiration to me. I did try to channel her a few times, especially the two occasions I posed for Horst, the photographer who had captured and immortalized her beauty so many times.

As much as I was drawn to Dietrich's toughness, I've always found Marilyn Monroe's vulnerability touching and her beauty irresistible. She never manifested strength and independence so I did not want to be like her, but her appearance was so desirable and genuine. I was just a young teenager in 1962 when she died of a drug overdose. I have collected portraits of Marilyn ever since.

Jackie Kennedy Onassis inspired me with her elegance, her beauty, and her incredible style. Style has so much to do with the way one handles oneself and I always admired Jackie's dignity at all moments of her tragic life. She never acted as a victim and always looked impeccable, even with bloodstains on the pink wool suit she refused to change out of the day her husband was killed. I was at boarding school in England then, and my mother had come to visit for the weekend. We watched the tragedy unfold on TV, sitting on our bed at the Hilton Hotel in London.

I remember meeting Jackie when Egon and I had dinner with her and her then husband, Greek tycoon Aristotle Onassis, at El Morocco in New York. She was as charming as he was rough. I hated the way he belittled her but I liked her enormously. I loved it when later, after he died, Jackie decided to have a private, ordinary life for herself and her kids in New York. She became an editor at the publishing house Doubleday. I remember the paparazzi photos of her walking the New York streets in her camel-colored pants and a sweater, with her trademark large, incognito sunglasses.

We lived one block from each other on Fifth Avenue where we were each raising two children on our own, a boy and a girl, although mine were much younger. My perfume Tatiana was her favorite. Later, one of her granddaughters would be named Tatiana. We shared the same hairdresser, Edgar. I identified with her in many ways, including our respective battles with cancer. Of all the women I admire, Jacqueline Bouvier Kennedy Onassis will truly remain the model of style, beauty, and courage.

Angelina Jolie is another woman I find both ravishing and interesting. I was attracted first by her free spirit and her unconventional life. I thought her desire to create a large family, adopting children from all sides of the world, was commendable. But it was when I saw the movie she wrote and directed about Bosnia, *In the Land of Blood and Honey*, that I began to truly admire her. I went to see the film on a rainy afternoon in Paris. Sitting by me were two Bosnian women, weeping. Angelina is continuing to address the huge issue of sexual violence in conflict and brought great attention to the cause. What makes Angelina uniquely beautiful is her substance and her wanting to give voice to those who have none.

Madonna was not what you would call a striking beauty when she appeared at a party in my apartment in the early eighties. She was nineteen years old and hiding under a huge dark felt hat. The only person who noticed her that night was my mother, with whom she talked for hours. What Madonna did have was personality, courage, ambition, and talent. She knew who she wanted to be. Her passion, her hard work, her constant desire to learn and improve, turned her into a great beauty, a superwoman, superstar, and role model, breaking boundaries and appealing to many generations. Madonna's personality created Madonna.

I had hoped to meet Mother Teresa in the 1970s when she came to New York and visited with Mayor Ed Koch. I found her strikingly beautiful and elegant in her white-and-blue-striped robe, full of humility, strength, love, and compassion. I was told she also had a lively sense of humor.

Another woman who personifies beauty, strength, and dignity is Oprah Winfrey. Oprah is simply the most formidable woman I've ever met. As a little girl, she knew she wanted a special life, so she defeated the huge obstacles she faced, worked incredibly hard, and became one of the world's most influential women. Oprah is bigger than life; she is life, all the good and purity of it. The strength of her desire to improve the world is a true example of beauty. I love her, respect her, and admire her, and feel so privileged to call her my friend.

I have been in awe of Gloria Steinem, who led the women's movement and improved our lives forever, since the moment I met her. Feminist and feminine, doer and dreamer, graceful, strong, and beautiful, her impact on the lives of all women is immeasurable. It is because of Gloria that I gave up using the title of princess and opted for Ms. It felt more glamorous at the time. Ms. meant freedom.

Character. Intelligence. Strength. Style. That makes beauty. All these attributes form beauty, and personality, that elusive state of being that is not necessarily perfect. "Beauty is perfect in its imperfections." It is our imperfections that make us different. Personality, not traditional beauty, is always what I've looked for in my models.

I was at a party in New York in 1970 when I saw this amazing-looking girl who was part of the court of Andy Warhol. She was very, very pale with an unusual face that looked like a mixture of Greta Garbo and a moonchild. She'd plucked off the ends of each of her eyebrows, which gave her a startled, almost comic expression—some said she looked like an exotic bug. She was about five foot six or so and weighed less than a hundred pounds—and looked different from everyone else.

I had just taken a showroom, my first, at the Gotham Hotel in New York for fashion week in April 1971 when I approached this seventeen-year-old. "Would you be interested in modeling my clothes to show buyers for a week?" I asked. "Sure," she said. And so Jane Forth became my first of many, many models.

I didn't know that I'd started a pattern that continues to this day: finding interesting-looking girls with personality at the very beginning of their lives and careers, girls I noticed because they were different. I'd found Jane just before she became famous—two months after fashion week, *Life* magazine did a four-page color spread of her titled "Just Plain Jane" that described her as "a new now face in the awesome tradition of Twiggy and Penelope Tree" and she starred in Andy's film *L'Amour*, which he wrote for her. I cannot claim that I discovered Jane or any of the other models who have worked for me over the years, but I do notice them very early on.

The models I hired for my second fashion show at the Pierre Hotel all became stars, as did the dress I was introducing for the first time—the wrap dress. The legends were born on an April afternoon, their names a future Who's Who of superstar models—Jerry Hall, Pat Cleveland, Apollonia. They also became my friends.

Apollonia was skinny, skinny, and tall as a beanstalk when she appeared for a go-see for the show. I'd never seen anyone so narrow and with such long legs. On top of that long body was a tiny head with a smiley, naughty face, and she spoke with a very strong Dutch accent (her last name was van Ravenstein). I liked her immediately. She had an amazing personality, kind and very funny and we became good friends. She worked for me many times on her way to becoming a top model in the seventies.

Pat Cleveland was a striking model, too, already well known by the time I started. She was a favorite of Stephen Burrows and Halston, the queen of the Halstonettes. Part black, part Cherokee, part Irish, Pat was unique and wonderfully flamboyant. She danced down the runway, moving her arms, her legs, and her derriere, living the clothes, embracing the music and taking the audience with her like a snake charmer. Pat also loved to sing, or was it lip-synching? I don't remember. What I do remember is that I always thought she was meant to play Josephine Baker, the spectacular black American performer who left America in the 1920s to establish herself as a megastar in France. Like Josephine, Pat was a real woman, bubbling with personality, and they looked very much alike. I tried to convince Barry to make a movie of Josephine Baker's life starring Pat, but it never went any further than my imagination.

At the same time I met Apollonia and Pat, Jerry Hall appeared on the New York scene and I used her as well for the show that launched the wrap dress. She, too, was very tall and very narrow; her six-foot frame seemed to be all legs. Jerry had huge blue eyes, flawless skin, and a cascade of long golden hair that she threw to one side like Rita Hayworth in the film *Gilda*. She was only seventeen, always accompanied by one of her many sisters. She laughed loudly and spoke with a very exotic Texas accent. She quickly became a major model and appeared on forty magazine covers in no time at all. She seduced the world and Mick Jagger, whom she subsequently married, and together they have four children.

Funny to think that so much stardom started on that April afternoon at the Cotillion Room of the Pierre Hotel . . . Jerry Hall, Pat Cleveland, Apollonia, and last but not least, the wrap dress!

I was doing a personal appearance at Lord & Taylor in New York in 1975 when I first saw this incredible Somali goddess coming up the escalator. "Who are you?" I asked, incredulous at such beauty and grace. She answered with a deep and secure voice: "My name is Iman, I've just arrived in New York and I am a model." When I asked for her phone number, she squatted on the floor to reach into the large basket she was carrying, looking for a pen and paper. Her magnificent body language and elegance were astounding. Squatting like that on the floor of a department store with her legs opened she could have been in a market in Mogadishu or a queen in a palace of a *Thousand and One Nights*. I was entranced.

Like many of the models I used, Iman was, and is, a strong, intelligent woman. She speaks five languages and went on to found a successful cosmetics and fashion company, establishing her own global brand. After one daughter and a divorce, she met and married the rock star David Bowie, with whom she shares another daughter and her life in New York. Iman has never forgotten her roots. She does important work for Raise Hope for Congo, UNICEF, Save the Children, and the Dr. Hawa Abdi Foundation.

Not all models have happy endings. I will always love Gia, whom I met at the Mudd Club in 1978. Dressed like a biker in a studded black leather jacket and cowboy boots, with no makeup, she was simply the most beautiful girl I'd ever seen. She was seventeen and doing a little modeling, she told me, having just arrived in New York from Pennsylvania. I was with Ara Gallant that night, and we both fell in love with her. To the best of my knowledge, I was the first to use her in an ad.

Gia was sassy and in your face—she loved to act as a bad boy, never wore makeup, and dressed often in men's clothes. Francesco Scavullo hired her to do *Cosmopolitan* covers, and later she worked with Richard Avedon, Arthur Elgort, and Chris von Wangenheim, the top photographers of the era.

She and I had a wonderful time together in 1979, when I hired her to do a campaign called "On the Eve of a New Decade." It incorporated all my products—clothes, perfume, intimate apparel, jeans. Chris von Wangenheim and I directed the whole shoot and I felt on top of the world. My business was booming. Gia was gorgeous. We laughed a lot and I adored her.

One weekend I invited her to come and join me in the Pines on Fire Island where Calvin Klein had loaned me his beach house with a striking black swimming pool. I was excited to see Gia. I had a girl's crush on her. She arrived, late, on a Saturday afternoon. I remember coming home after a long walk on the beach to find her inexplicably sitting on the floor of the bedroom closet. She became agitated and embarrassed when she saw me. I did not understand what was going on then, but looking back, I think she was probably shooting up; I found out later she had become a serious heroin addict.

A few months after that weekend, Gia came to my office in dirty clothes looking gaunt. She needed cash. Even though I knew what she "needed" it for, I could not refuse her and gave her what was in my wallet. I never saw her again. It was probably from a dirty needle that she contracted AIDS and died in 1986 at the age of twenty-six.

A very young Angelina Jolie starred in the HBO film of Gia's troubled life. For years I couldn't watch it. Recently I did and was astounded by how accurate and real the movie was.

Years after Gia's death, I was asked to be part of a documentary about her. I went to some studio on the West Side to do the interview. It was important to me that people know what a lovely, generous woman Gia was. As I was about to leave the studio, I met Gia's mother, herself a very beautiful woman, who had also come to be interviewed. I hugged her and felt close to her. She surprised me by telling me that after her daughter's death, she had found a sealed letter from Gia addressed to me. When I smiled, she immediately added, "I opened it, read it, but will never give it to you." I was hurt and confused by that comment, and I wish I knew what Gia had written.

There were so many other wonderful models that I worked with along the way. Cindy Crawford, who looked like Gia, though she turned her beauty into a happy, healthy family life. Patti Hansen, the rock 'n' roll girl who ended up marrying bad boy genius Keith Richards and had two hip, rock 'n' roll daughters with him; French beauty Inès de la Fressange whom I used in 1982 before she became a muse for Karl Lagerfeld at Chanel; Rene Russo, who became a movie star. I then stopped working for a while, and never used any of the supermodels who appeared on the scene and who I admired from afar . . . Linda Evangelista, Claudia Schiffer, Christy Turlington, Stella Tennant, and Stephanie Seymour.

Though I did not have a runway for her to walk down at the time, I couldn't resist meeting Naomi Campbell. By then Barry had taken over QVC, the TV home shopping network, and I was acting as a talent recruiter. I wanted Naomi to go on it. I remember inviting her to lunch at the Four Seasons in New York. Everyone stared at her as she walked into the front, "power" room. She looked like a goddess. We talked about everything but TV shopping. I never brought it up. She was too fresh, too good for it. We stayed friends and worked together a few times and she showed up for me big time with her powerful Russian then fiancé when I had my first exhibition in Moscow years later. She came through again, a huge surprise, on the runway for my Spring 2014 collection. The crowd burst into cheers as the incomparable supermodel appeared to close the show.

I never worked with the biggest model of the decade, Kate Moss, but she is my kind of girl: true to herself, independent, and in charge of her own life. When I met her at a photography opening in London, she told me, "I want to grow up to be you." I answered promptly, "You already are, my dear!" We were both flattered.

Natalia Vodianova caught my attention immediately when she first came to New York in 2001 at the age of nineteen. I was drawn to her freshness and determination and felt her strength and her character as soon as I met her. She opened and closed my show. It was her first, I think, in New York. Soon after that she became a top international model and a close friend. Her strength, I learned, had been born out of hardship. Her father had left her mother when she was a toddler, and they were impoverished. She was only nine when she started selling fruit with her mother on the street in Gorky to help support her two half sisters, one of whom was born with cerebral palsy and deeply autistic.

I was in my office in September 2004 when Natalia came to me in tears. Masked terrorists had taken an entire school in Beslan, Russia, and held everyone hostage. Three hundred and thirty-four people were killed, among them at least 186 children. The children who survived suffered emotional trauma, burns, and other injuries.

"We've got to do something for the children," Natalia said. "Help me to raise money." We gave a fund-raising party in my studio on West Twelfth Street. She was so young then, so inexperienced, yet within days she had orchestrated the entire event: an ice palace décor, a vodka sponsorship, celebrities and paparazzi and a full charity auction that raised hundreds of thousands of dollars.

She created her own foundation, Naked Heart, that has built over a hundred play parks in areas of Russia where there were none so children can have a place to be safe. Now her organization has expanded its work to provide support to families raising children with special needs throughout Russia.

In February 2008, I had the wild idea to put her together with my longtime friend, French writer, photographer, and artist François-Marie Banier, to create an ad campaign. I had always admired François-Marie, first for his novels and plays in the seventies, and recently for his extraordinary photographs. I called him in Paris and arranged for him to meet Natalia. A few weeks later they came to New York.

"Make magic," I told them, and magic happened. They walked the streets of the Meatpacking District and he photographed her with wet hair and no makeup in front of walls covered with colorful graffiti, then painted on the photos and decorated them with endless stream-of-consciousness writings. It was quite a rebellious campaign. You could not see the clothes at all, just a beautiful woman tattooed with splashes of color and writings. It was art and the only thing that indicated they were ads was the logo, DVF. I'm not sure those images were commercially understood, but I was thrilled when, at a party in Paris, Karl Lagerfeld congratulated me on the boldness of the campaign. I was very proud that the "magic" collaboration I'd thought of was later published by Steidl in a beautiful art book.

Because I know how to bring out a woman's strength and make her feel confident, and because I have become skilled at photography, I have, along the way, taken memorable photos of women. I photographed the ravishing, exotic, French/Italian/Egyptian Elisa Sednaoui for *V* magazine; the Colombian politician, activist, and FARC prisoner of seven years, Ingrid Betancourt, for the art magazine *Egoïste*; and did a full fashion story for the French magazine *CRASH*. I enjoyed making those women feel the strongest and the most desirable they had ever felt. Last but not least, I loved that process with our family's own gorgeous Alison Kay, mother of my fourth grandchild, Leon. We did two DVF advertising campaigns together. She is as beautiful outside as I know her to be inside.

Casting for a fashion show is very different from choosing a model to advertise your brand. Each time we cast a show, we hire a stylist and a casting agent. They know all the best girls and call a "go-see." I am often amazed how plain and unassuming some of the new top girls look in real life, and how you need a special eye to recognize a strange face that can become beautiful, an unusual bone structure that catches the light, an oddness that becomes magical. Every casting takes me back to an episode decades ago, in Geneva, Switzerland, when I was briefly a receptionist at IOS, the "Fund of Funds" company created by financier Bernard Cornfeld.

Bernie was a friend of Jerry Ford, the founder, with his wife, Eileen, of the Ford model agency in New York, and Jerry was visiting the IOS office. As he was waiting in the reception area, he went by the desk of the other receptionist and handed her his card. "If you ever want to model," he said, "let me know. You have potential." I was shocked and offended. Why her and not me? I certainly thought I was more interesting than that pale, tall, very plain skinny girl, but it turned out that it was precisely because she was that white canvas of a woman that he thought she could make an interesting model. I have thought about it at every one of my castings since.

Runway models don't move the way they used to. Unlike Pat Cleveland who danced down the runway, they are taught to march like soldiers without a smile. I always surprise my own models when just before the show I tell them, "Smile, seduce, and be you. Be the woman you want to be!" I believe I am one of the very few designers who ask their models to smile. Joie de vivre is very much on brand at DVF.

My definition of beauty is strength and personality. Strength is captivating: the women I've seen in India working the fields in their orange saris, their arms covered with colorful glass bangles; the women working in construction in Indonesia, carrying heavy bricks on their heads; the women carrying their children to bush hospitals in Africa.

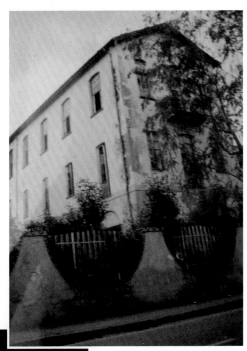

Manifattura Tessile
Ferretti in Parè, Como.

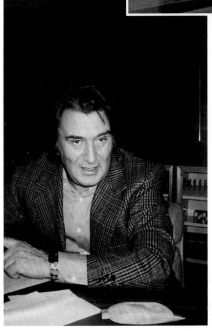

My friend and mentor
Angelo Ferretti.

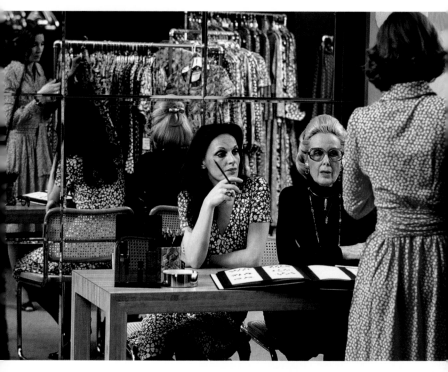

In my 7th Avenue showroom in 1976. *(Burt Glinn, Magnum)*

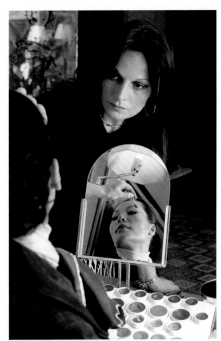

Applying makeup on a customer. *(Burt Glinn, Magnum)*

Working on Tatiana fragrance products, 1976.
(Elliot Erwitt, Magnum)

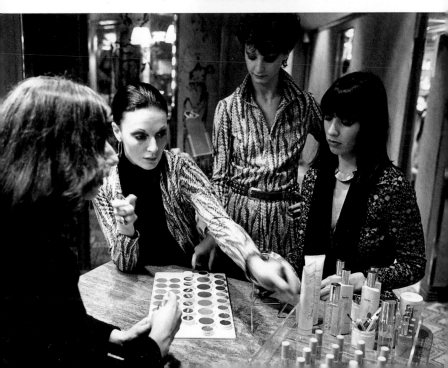

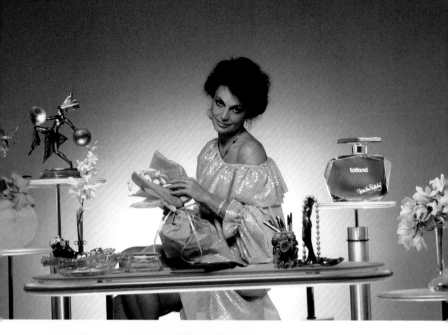

TV commercial for Tatiana fragrance, 1982. *(Albert Watson)*

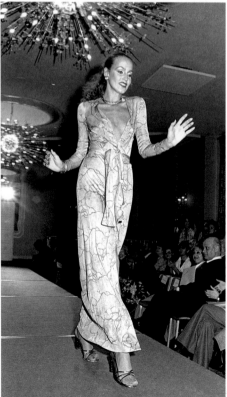

A teenage Jerry Hall on the runway at the Pierre hotel in 1975. *(Nick Machalaba, Corbis Image)*

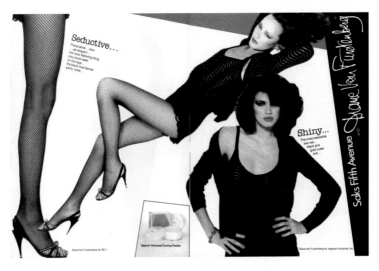

Gia Carangi for Diane von Furstenberg ad campaign, 1979. *(Chris von Wangenheim)*

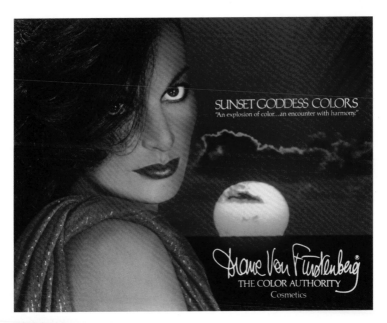

Ad campaign for the Color Authority cosmetics line in 1982. *(Albert Watson)*

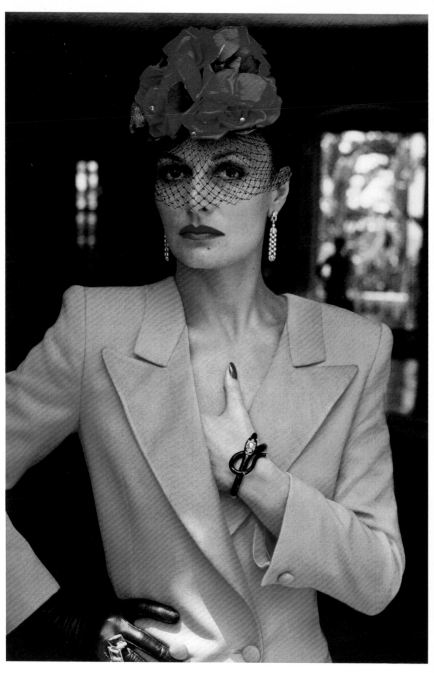

Photographed by Helmut Newton for the advertising
campaign for the couture line. *(© The Helmut Newton Estate)*

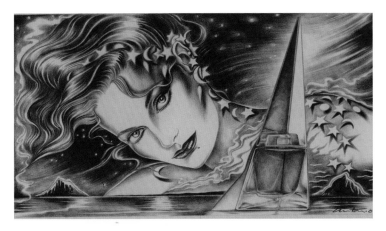

An illustration by Antonio Lopez for
Volcan d'Amour perfume. *(Artwork by Antonio Lopez)*

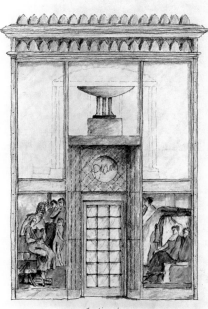

Architect Michael Graves's
sketch for the Diane
couture boutique at the
Sherry-Netherland hotel.
*(Drawing by Michael Graves,
courtesy of Michael Graves &
Associates)*

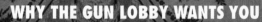
WHY THE GUN LOBBY WANTS YOU

LEAR'S

JANUARY 1994 $3.00

**POST-HOLIDAY
PAMPERING**
At-Home
Spa Treatments

**WASHINGTON
WOMEN**
An Inside-the-Beltway
Guide to Pols,
Pundits, and
Other Players

**LETTERS TO
MY EX-HUSBAND**

PERFECT PITCH
DIANE VON FURSTENBERG
and the Retail Revolution

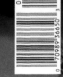

PLUS: Nanci Griffith • Serious Stretching • Vest Bets
Tuition Terror • Gabriel Byrne • John Guare

Cover of *Lear's* magazine in my QVC days, 1994. *(Michel Arnaud, courtesy of the artist)*

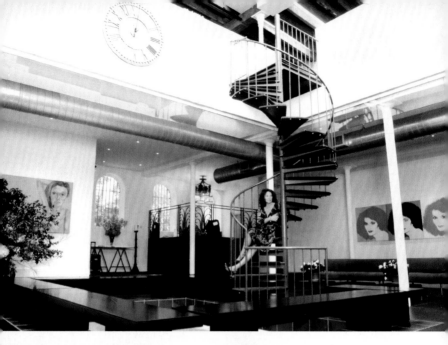

Inside of DVF Studio on West 12th Street. *(Emanuele Scorcelletti, courtesy of the artist)*

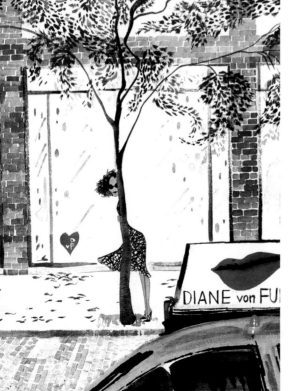

Ruben Toledo's illustration of the first shop on West 12th Street. *(Artwork by Ruben Toledo)*

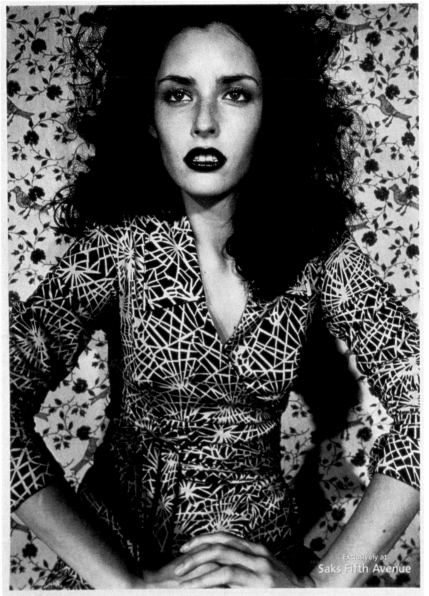

Exclusively at
Saks Fifth Avenue

He stared at me all night. Then he said...

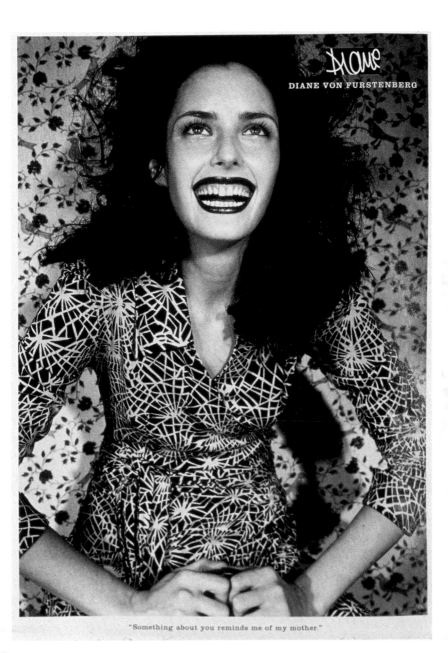

"Something about you reminds me of my mother."

Model Daniela photographed by Bettina Rheims for the wrap
dress relaunch, 1997. *(Bettina Rheims, courtesy of the artist)*

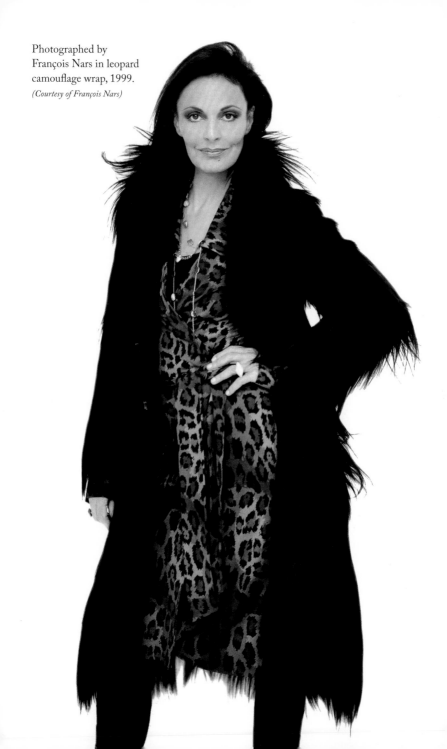

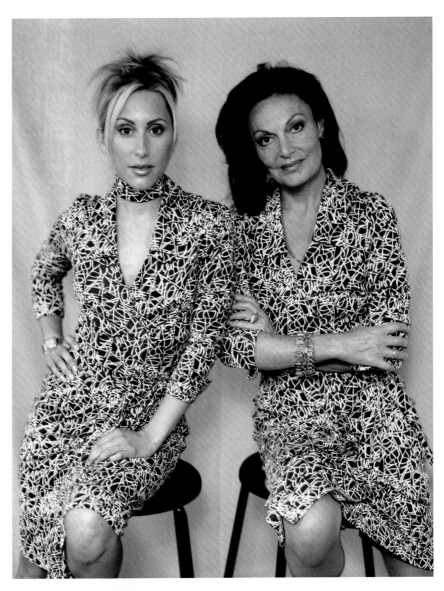

Wrap for a new generation. With daughter-in-law,
Alexandra, in 1998. *(Steffen Thalemann)*

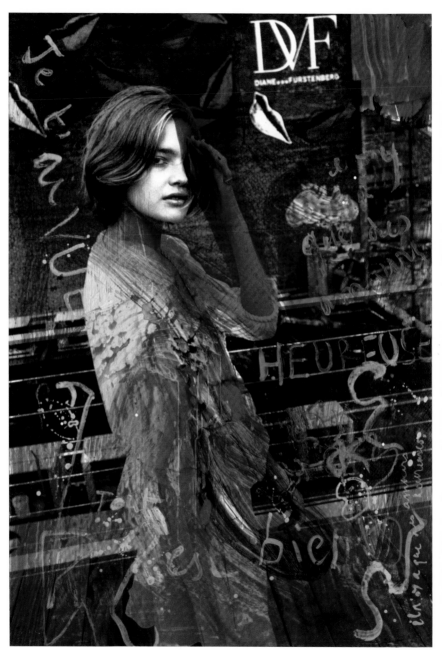

Natalia Vodianova photographed and painted by François-Marie Banier, 2008.

(François-Marie Banier, courtesy of the artist)

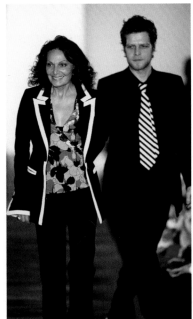

Walking the runway
with creative director
Nathan Jenden, 2002.
(Dan Lecca)

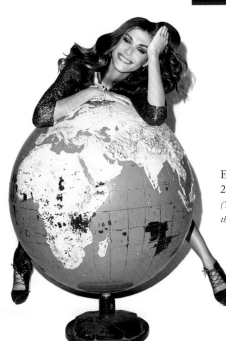

Elisa Sednaoui for the
2011 DVF campaign.
*(Terry Richardson, courtesy of
the artist)*

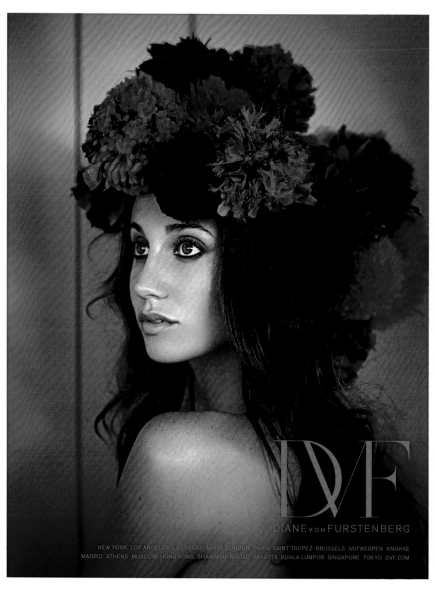

Ali Kay photographed by me for the 2010 DVF campaign.

The dignity of these women with their innate elegance is a true inspiration of beauty.

Some of the strongest women I know are the women of Vital Voices, a global nonprofit originally founded by Hillary Clinton when she was First Lady, on whose board I sit. Vital Voices identifies women leaders from around the world and helps them to increase their leadership potential. I've been both humbled and inspired by these women who not only have survived their own misery, but are committed to helping others in their communities.

Women like tiny, four-foot-six Sunitha Krishnan, who was gang-raped by eight men at fifteen and went on to form an organization in India called Prajwala that rescues and rehabilitates girls from brothels and sex traffickers. Sunitha has been beaten up and regularly receives death threats, but perseveres, harnessing what she calls "the power of pain." You barely notice Sunitha, she is so small, but once she starts speaking, she becomes so beautiful and majestic.

And Dr. Kakenya Ntaiya, a Kenyan who was engaged to be married at five and later bartered with her father to be circumcised in return for the opportunity to go to high school. Kakenya went on to college and graduate school in the US and returned to her Masai village to establish a girls' boarding school that changed the direction of education in her country.

And Chouchou Namegabe, a young journalist from the Democratic Republic of Congo who recorded the stories of hundreds of voiceless rape victims and played them on the radio to try to shame the government into taking action, then testified on behalf of the women at the International Court in the Hague.

These are but a few of the many women I've met through Vital Voices who have left me almost breathless with their courage and determination. "My God," I think to myself. "I've done nothing." Though

I've dedicated myself to empowering women through my work in fashion, mentoring, and philanthropy, *I* am empowered, mentored, and filled with riches from these women. It is they, and many others like them, who inspire me with their strength and beauty.

One day, after hearing me talk so much about Vital Voices, my children had an idea: "You are always talking about these Vital Voices women. You're so inspired by them; you should give them awards. The family foundation can sponsor them—we can help finance their work."

That idea stayed in the back of my mind, but it was unresolved until my friend Tina Brown, editor then of The Daily Beast, asked me to join her in organizing the first Women in the World Summit: three days of the most powerful women meeting, talking, and coming up with solutions for global challenges. I was so excited to be involved in this conference and it felt natural to turn one evening into a big dinner at the United Nations, and give awards, each with a $50,000 grant.

And that is how the DVF Awards were established in 2010 by the Diller–von Furstenberg Family Foundation to honor and support extraordinary women who have had the courage to fight, the power to survive, and the leadership to inspire; women who have transformed the lives of others through their commitment, resources, and visibility. Since 2010, we have honored so many inspiring and truly beautiful women, among them women from the Vital Voices network. We have also honored Hillary Clinton; Oprah Winfrey; Robin Roberts, anchor of ABC's *Good Morning America*; and Gloria Steinem with Lifetime Leadership Awards. Ingrid Betancourt, Elizabeth Smart, and Jaycee Dugard have received Inspiration Awards. What these three women have in common is that they were all kidnapped and, like my mother, held in harrowing captivity, and, like her, refuse to think of themselves as victims. "My hope is to be remembered for what I do, and not what happened to me," said Jaycee, who was held for eighteen years and has since founded the JAYC Foundation, which helps families recover from abduction and other trauma.

We also established a People's Voice Award, chosen by popular vote from four nominees who are working within the United States. They are women who all start in a small grassroots way. As my mother told me, if you save one life, it begins a dynasty. The life you save can save another, so one life is never too small.

Bravery and determination: that is also beauty.

———

Beauty is health and health is beauty. That is the reminder I email, as president of the Council of Fashion Designers of America to designers every season before their shows. When I was elected president of the trade organization in 2006, there was a lot in the press about the causes of anorexia and its prevalence in young girls. I had no personal experience with eating disorders for myself or my daughter or anyone close to me. So I was puzzled at first when I was told that the fashion industry was complicit in the rise in eating disorders.

I was naïve, perhaps. Many top models have become celebrities so it would be natural for young girls to want to emulate them. Still, starving themselves was not the answer. Long, thin bodies are genetic, not engineered. Models watch what they eat, of course, but for the most part, their bodies are predisposed to be thin. This can be difficult for young girls to accept.

Though becoming a model is a dream for many all over the world, the truth is it is not an easy job. More often than not it is about being rejected, about feeling bad about yourself. Most of the top agencies mean well and are caring for the girls—some are even outstandingly protective—but there are pseudoagencies and there is trafficking and prostitution that happens "in the name of fashion." I cannot warn girls enough to be vigilant. Don't dream of becoming a model unless it is genuinely possible. Look for other doors. The business of beauty can often be anything but beautiful.

In fact, I plead with young girls, except the very few genetically exceptional ones, not to try and become models. "Use your brains, your common sense and do not become an object," I told one graduating high school class. "The way you look is important, but who you are and how you project it is eventually who you will become and how you will appear."

I became convinced that the CFDA had to take the initiative to promote health as beauty. We established industry standards in 2007, working in partnership with medical experts, modeling agencies, and *Vogue* editor in chief Anna Wintour. These standards include commonsense recommendations to protect the girls; workshops for designers, models, and their families on how to recognize the signs of eating disorders; and encouraging models with eating disorders to seek professional help.

Next we addressed age. Youth is a huge factor in the business of fashion and the age issue is a stubborn and long-standing one—for many, the younger the better. It is a hard battle because many designers think clothes look better on very tall, extremely skinny girls, and the younger they are, the less formed they are. Those designers influence the bookers and force the model agencies to supply girls who are younger and younger. We had to stop that downward spiral, or at least slow it down. Every member of the CFDA—the top 450 designers in America—is now required to check a runway model's ID to ensure that she is at least sixteen and that those under eighteen are not kept at work past midnight at fittings or photo shoots. Health is beauty. Beauty is health.

———————

I was diagnosed with cancer in 1994, at the age of forty-seven. One minute I was fine, the next I was undergoing radiation at the base of my tongue and soft palette. It started at a lunch with Ralph Lauren at the famous midtown New York restaurant La Grenouille. It was supposed to be a business lunch but we talked about everything, including love and the fragility of life. He had recently had a benign tumor removed from his brain, he said. "How did you find out you had the tumor?" I asked. "I kept hearing some noise in my left ear." As he said those words I heard a noise in my left ear. The following day it was still there. Could it be my imagination? I made an appointment with an ear doctor.

"There is nothing wrong with your ear," the doctor told me, but he found a swollen gland on the right side of my neck. He didn't seem concerned and gave me antibiotics. The noise disappeared but the swelling did not. I then had a biopsy and nothing bad came out. "It is a benign cyst, don't worry," I was told. I did not like the idea of having a cyst, so I scheduled a surgical procedure to have it removed the following week, on Friday, May 13. The unlucky date proved prophetic. As I woke up groggy from the anesthesia with Tatiana and my mother by my side, the doctor told us the news. When they removed the cyst, they had cut it in half and found tiny, tiny bad squamous cancerous cells that had already metastasized. Tatiana was shocked. My mother thought she'd misunderstood what she'd heard so she turned to Tatiana and kept insisting, "Translate for me! Tell me in French!"

The following days were terrifying, going for all kinds of tests and fearing the worst. An operation that would cut most of my neck away? Chemotherapy? Everything sounded scary. It did not help when I went home the night of my diagnosis and turned on the news to hear that Jackie Kennedy Onassis had died of cancer that day.

At first I felt in the dark and very worried, but little by little, as I understood better what the doctors were explaining to me, I regained my strength and pushed away the fear. I had to accept that I had cancer and deal with it. Seven weeks of radiation. An unexpected summer was suddenly laid out in front of me. It was going to be a time of treatment and healing. I had no choice but to accept it, take time for myself, and focus on my health. I had to get well, kill the bad cells forever, and never, ever let them come back. I repeated that sentence over and over to myself so often that it became a little victory song in French.

My mother stayed by me. She did not act worried, which gave me strength. Alexandre returned from Hong Kong where he had been working at a bank; Tatiana was nearby. Barry was hit hard by the news. My doctor told me he saw him walking to his car the day I was diagnosed and never had he seen someone's posture reveal so much distress.

On my first weekend in Connecticut after the diagnosis, my friend, producer, and agent Sandy Gallin, gave me a life-changing gift. He sent Deepak Chopra, the famous Indian New Age doctor and author, to visit me at Cloudwalk. We sat together as he taught me how to meditate. His way of explaining things reached me, reassured me, and turned out to be extremely helpful. He invited me to the Chopra Center for Wellbeing in La Jolla, California, and I went before starting the radiation. Tatiana took me there and spent the first two days with me, but I needed to be alone. I meditated and repeated the sutras Deepak gave me: Peace, Harmony, Laughter, Love, Creativity, Affluence,

Abundance, Discrimination, Integration, Freedom, Truth, Knowledge, Infinity, Immortality, Enlightenment, Holiness. I walked on the beach for hours, swam hundreds of laps in the pool, and had long conversations with myself and God. All of that plus the Ayurveda treatments of diet, herbs, and massage, along with the calmness around me, helped prepare me for this unexpected battle.

Back in New York, Alexandre took me to an appointment where they made measurements for a mask and put tiny tattoos on my face to ensure the rays would aim precisely. Years later my doctor told me Alexandre had returned to him after walking me out to ask him to take special care of me, "Remember: it's my mother you're dealing with."

I took a photo of my face in the bathroom mirror before I went to my first radiation session. I wanted to remember me as I was, not knowing if I'd be changed forever. And then the routine began. Every day I walked to Sloan Kettering and put on the mask that was attached to the table. For thirty seconds, the rays targeted each side of my neck and the middle. I would then start walking home to the Carlyle Hotel, stop to have wheat grass juice at the health food store (it was nauseating, but I believed in its natural healing powers), and then walk on singing my little French victory song to kill the bad cells. At home, I meditated for hours, had a daily massage to stimulate the immune system, and gargled with sesame oil. On the weekend, when there were no treatments, I went to Cloudwalk and enjoyed the beauty of nature—the forest, the flowers, the deer among the apple trees. Nature had never felt more beautiful, more peaceful, and more reassuring.

Deepak called every day. So did Egon from Italy, Mark Peploe from London, and my friends from all over the world. I felt loved without being pitied and serene from the strength that comes from love. Barry started to talk about us living together, getting a house, and started inquiring about my relationship with Mark, which he'd never done before. I was vague. My future was uncertain; I did not know what I wanted except to get well.

In the middle of the treatment my friend Mort Zuckerman, the real estate tycoon, invited me to go to the White House for a state dinner the president and Mrs. Clinton were giving for the emperor and the empress of Japan. I was excited and accepted. The grand master fashion designer of the moment, John Galliano, happened to be doing his first personal appearance at Bergdorf Goodman across the street from my office, and I borrowed his most beautiful ball gown: pale pink and blue chiffon, with lots of ruffles and a long train that went on forever. In spite of the radiation burn shadings on each side of my face, which I managed to hide with makeup, I ended up looking beautiful as I walked into the tented Rose Garden. The dinner was a historic event and I really enjoyed being there. At my table were some important Japanese businesspeople who could not believe that they actually were in the same room as their emperor. In Japan, they would have had to be separated by a screen because no common subjects can be in the same room with his Excellency the Emperor!

For me it was a different kind of excitement. I loved my voluptuous dress, though I had to shuffle carefully with my long train that nonetheless was stepped on by everybody and ended up in shreds by the end of the evening. Feeling frivolous and beautiful in the middle of my painful treatment was a wink to myself. It felt great.

The news from Belgium, however, was not good. Philippe phoned me just before the Fourth of July. My father's health was failing; we had to get ready for the worst. The radiation center in New York was closed for a few days over the holiday weekend and Barry generously gave me his plane to visit my father. By then, I had lost all sense of taste, my throat was hurting, and my skin was very burned, but I had to see my father. His Alzheimer's had taken a bad turn and I knew he would no longer recognize me. Still, I wanted to kiss him and thank him for the love he had given me. Tatiana came with me. It was the last time we saw him.

On the way back from Belgium, we landed in Gander, Canada, to refuel. It had been raining and the plane sat between two complete rainbows. Tatiana told me to make a wish. I wished to be cured. There were another dozen daily treatments left to go, a dryer throat, and more burns. Deepak kept on calling, my mother, Barry, and the children were nearby, and I was counting the days. It was the year of the World Cup. Brazil won, and I did, too.

I went back to Deepak's center in California after the treatments to recuperate. That was the worst week of all. As my doctor had predicted, the discomfort increased. I was burned inside and out from the radiation and exhausted. The adrenaline that had sustained me during treatment was gone because I knew the treatments were over. I locked myself in my room and moaned. The only thing I forced myself to do was fifty laps in the pool, repeating my sutras.

At the end of the week, a call came in the middle of the night, morning in Brussels. My father had passed away. My brother and my mother were on the phone, crying. My eyes stayed dry; my father was gone forever and there was nothing I could do to change that. On the plane from La Jolla, I picked up Alexandre in Las Vegas and we flew to New York and then on to Belgium. Tatiana met us at the Brussels airport—she had come from Portugal. We went straight to my father's apartment, the apartment I grew up in. His room seemed smaller than I remembered; the coffin seemed small, too. I sat by it. On the side table there was a lit candle and photos of my father's parents and brother. I felt helpless but peaceful, thankful for the love my father had given me. We buried him in a lovely cemetery, surrounded by trees and stillness. The children left that afternoon. I needed a break. I decided to go to Berlin for a long weekend and meet Mark, who was there editing his movie *Victory*. My brother thought I was too weak to travel, but I wanted to feel life and love, so I went. I rested in my hotel room during the day while Mark was working, but at night we walked around the streets of the newly united Berlin and loved it.

A few days later, I went back to Brussels to tidy up my father's home. Like me, he had kept everything: diaries, letters, photographs ... memory lane in all its splendor. I missed his presence, his smell, but in the mirror I could see him—our features are so similar. Before leaving, I took his favorite watch, a gold Omega, his crocodile wallet, and his two Russian glasses with silver holders in which he drank his tea every day.

Confronting my cancer was challenging, but enriching. I became more compassionate to the sufferings of others, appreciated the value of health, became more spiritual and understood both my fragility and my strength. I have been thankful ever since to God, the doctors, my family, my friends, and my own power. My little French song worked and I have been cancer-free ever since.

I became much more health conscious after my bout with cancer. I eat lightly and in moderation—fresh, organic vegetables and fruits, grains and beans, little meat—and I resist sugar as much as I'm able to, but I still love dark chocolate and an occasional glass of great red wine. I drink lots of water—lots—and cups of hot, fresh ginger tea with lemon and honey.

My legs are stronger than they were when I was thirty because of all the hikes I love to do. Uphill, the steeper the better. The Appalachian Trail winds through the hills near Cloudwalk on its way from Maine to Georgia, and Barry, Shannon, and I hike on sections of it every day we are there. In LA we meet the children between our homes, at the bottom of Franklin Canyon, and hike to the peak together. When we're on the boat, we hike on whatever island or coast we pull into. I lead the way because I am faster. We are silent going up. Hiking is a meditation of sorts to me and I use it as a time to go within myself and enjoy the effort of climbing and the beauty of nature. We linger at the top, enjoying our accomplishment, and Barry leads the way down. That's when we talk, often our best talks, because of the long silence of the climb and the space that nature has given our minds to get clearer. I love those moments.

When I'm in New York, I climb up and down the five flights of stairs at the DVF headquarters, sometimes taking the steps two at a time, even in high heels. I swim just as strenuously, whether in the sea, the pool at Cloudwalk, or any hotel I stay at around the world. It is also a meditation. Exercising and counting the lengths crowd all thoughts out of the brain and I'm alone with myself.

I stay supple by doing yoga a couple of times a week in the yoga studio I built in a room next to my office. The stretching and the twists make me aware of every part of my body and keep me very flexible. Deep breathing is an integral part of yoga and I practice the long inhale and slow exhale to ease stressful moments. I also have a facial once a week from an Englishwoman named Tracie Martyn who attaches something, I don't know what, to her fingertips, which channels low-voltage electricity to my face and helps fight gravity. (So does smiling, I learned from fashion photographer Mario Testino.) I've been going to Tracie for fifteen years now, and my office knows it's the only appointment that can't be canceled.

Most important, I have a massage at least once a week, especially when I'm traveling. I used to think massages were vain and indulgent, but I've learned that isn't true. Massage bolsters the body's defense system, aids circulation, and rids your body of toxins.

While I was undergoing the cancer treatments, I started a weekly Shiatsu session. (I also have deep-tissue massages from Andrey, an excellent Ukrainian masseur.) My wonderful Shiatsu practitioner, who unexpectedly died of a stroke last year, was a talented Japanese man named Eizo who also healed the radiation blisters in my mouth by giving me a powder from a rare mushroom. He worked on me for nineteen years, every Tuesday morning before Tracie Martyn, giving me a deep-tissue massage to correct disharmonies and walking up and down my back to crack me. I miss him dearly.

Another result of my encounter with cancer is Dr. Durrafourd, a homeopathic doctor in Paris that my friend actress Marisa Berenson introduced me to. I see him once a year. He does full blood work, calculates the results, and prescribes me all kinds of antioxidants—all plant-based and natural. I have a dozen little bottles of pills and some liquids, which I keep together in a bag that I carry with me around the world. Have they had a positive effect? I like to think so. I went through menopause easily, for example. One day I stopped having my period and that was it.

Marisa also introduced me to Bianca, a healer who was able to ease the discomfort of my burns. I still call her in moments of crisis. I am the godmother of her son, Julien.

What I have learned is that when you are sick, much of healing is in the hands of doctors and science, but part of it is finding and using your own power.

Aging is out of your control. How you handle it, though, is in your hands.

When I was a girl, I always wanted to be older than I was. Instead of sitting, I knelt next to my father in the car so that people would think I was a grown-up. I pretended I had wrinkles and scratched my face with my nails because I wanted to have a lived-in face like the French movie star Jeanne Moreau. When I turned twenty and my mother asked me, "How does it feel being twenty?" I said, "Well, I've been telling people I've been twenty for so long that it doesn't make a difference." I always looked older than my actual years, so much so that when *Newsweek* put me on the cover on March 22, 1976, the editors didn't believe I was twenty-nine and sent a reporter to the Brussels town hall to check my birth certificate.

I had started my adult life at twenty-two, had two children by the time I was twenty-four, and a successful financial life by thirty. Looking back, I realize I was pretty in my late twenties, but I didn't really think so. I knew how to enhance what I had, highlighting my eyes and cheekbones, playing with my hair and my legs and acting with confidence. I knew I was seductive, but I never thought I was beautiful.

My thirties were my best years. I was still young but felt grown up, lived an adventurous life, raised my two children, and ran a business. I was independent and felt very free. I had total complicity with myself and my looks and I felt in charge. I had become the woman I wanted to be.

The forties were harder. My children went off to boarding school and college, and I sold my business. I was not sure who I was or who I wanted to be anymore. I went in and out of looks and started to question my own style. When I lost my fashion business, I lost the way of expressing myself creatively. I also had my battle with cancer.

Things got better when I hit fifty. I went back to work, creating a new studio environment and repositioning my brand. I surrounded myself with a new generation of girls. I was again the woman I wanted to be . . . engaged and engaging. I married Barry and became a grandmother. I embraced my age and my life. It was the beginning of the age of fulfillment, which continues. Now, in my sixties, I know I have less time ahead and want to enjoy, enjoy as much as possible.

I'm grateful I never thought of myself as beautiful when I was young. We all fade somewhat as time goes on. Women who relied only on their beauty can feel invisible later in life. It's a pity, for I feel in the latter part of your life you should feel fulfilled, not defeated. My advice is that as a woman gets deep into her forties, she should start becoming a myth. To become a myth for whatever she does, even if it's making the best chocolate mousse or being the best flower arranger. She has to stand for something and she's got to stay relevant, to be active, to participate. That's why I think it's so important for women to have an identity outside the home.

And never, ever lie about your age. Who can lie with the Internet anyway? To embrace your age is to embrace your life. Lying about your age, or about anything for that matter, is the beginning of trouble; it is the beginning of lying about who you are. What is important is to live fully every single day of every period of every age so that no time gets wasted. Because the time goes by, faster and faster.

So much of physical beauty is youth, pure and simple. The skin is fresh and tight, the eyes clear and wide, the waist slimmer, the hair full and lush, even the teeth, white and unworn. I never understood that as a girl. When somebody told me that I looked fresh, I hated it and found it unappealing. It's only when you stop being fresh that you appreciate it.

Youth is wonderful; it's exciting because it is the beginning of life. Everything is ahead and there is nothing more thrilling than beginnings when everything is possible and you can dream big dreams. But every day is a beginning. Living and enjoying the present moment to its fullest is the best way, the only way, to approach life. It is essential to learn from the past and look into the future without resentment. Resentments are toxic and can only pollute the future.

The best thing about aging, I have come to understand, is that you have a past. No one can take that away, so you'd better like it. That is why it is so important to waste no time. By living fully every day, you create your life and that becomes your past, a rich past.

When I was very young, I was arrogant and used to boast that I'd retire at thirty. As I got older, I continued to be arrogant about my age, but in a different way. I defied it. I would be dismissive and say, "Oh, age means nothing."

Today my energy has yet to let me down and I am more engaged than ever. But I am not as dismissive about it as I realize that aging can make you feel vulnerable. Perhaps it was a ski accident I had at the start of 2011 that made me more humble. One minute I'd been skiing happily with Barry in Aspen, Colorado; the next minute I was flat on my back in the snow with my face bleeding.

It had been a spectacular, sunny day on the mountain and I was skiing well and carefully between my ski instructor and Barry, and avoiding all of the aggressive snowboarders. My friend the actress Natasha Richardson had died the year before in a freak ski accident and she was very much on my mind when suddenly, out of nowhere,

came an out-of-control first-time skier. I was standing still, waiting for
Barry, when he hit me! He barreled into me with such force that he
left my face bloody and numb.

After an X-ray in Aspen showed my ribs were fractured and my
nose was broken, we flew to LA to have an MRI of my face to make
sure the eye orbit bones were not broken as well, which would have
required immediate surgery. In the plane I kept touching my cheekbones, terrified they were broken; they are my face's best asset. Luckily
there were only hairline fractures around my eyes that would heal and
the cheekbones were fine, but my mangled face set off alarms when we
got to the hospital. I felt that everyone I saw in the corridors thought I
was a victim of domestic abuse. It is amazing how quickly you can feel
like a victim and I felt that I had to justify my bruised face to everyone
who passed by. "Ski accident," I kept repeating. "Ski accident."

The timing of the accident couldn't have been worse. I had a
couple of big months coming up—a photo shoot that week, the acceptance of a huge award at a gala benefit for amFAR (Foundation for
AIDS Research) in New York, my Fall runway show during fashion
week, and a high-profile trip to China in the spring where an exten-
sive retrospective of my life and work was being installed in Beijing's
prestigious Pace Gallery. It was because of that very busy schedule
ahead of me that Barry had rented a house in Aspen for just the two
of us for a few days.

Immediately after the MRI, the doctor mentioned surgery. I was
not quite sure what he had in mind, but I said no. I wanted my face to
heal completely first and then see what needed to be done. From that
moment on, it was all about ice and arnica, arnica and ice. Very slowly
the swelling went down to reveal dark blue bruises that spread downward, creating a devastating expression. Arnica and more arnica slowly

lightened the color from dark purple to a lighter shade of purple, lavender, and eventually, weeks later, yellow. I recorded the progress daily on my iPhone; I had taken the first photo immediately after the fall and sent it to all of my friends. I continued to document the map of my face every day for the next two months. "This is what I look like," I would say to myself, "and it is not pretty."

I was still so bruised two weeks later that I considered passing up the amFAR benefit where I was going to be honored together with President Bill Clinton. I dreaded showing my face publicly, but then I felt ashamed for being so frivolous. "What are a few bruises compared to AIDS?" I scolded myself. "Of course you have to go."

Still, to partially cover my face, I asked my art department to make me a little fan. They made it heart-shaped, inscribed with my motto: "Love is life is love is life." I hid behind it at the beginning of the evening, but as soon as I went up onstage to accept the award, I put it down and simply said, "Excuse my appearance, I had a ski accident."

I didn't hide my face again. I wore sunglasses to my fashion show, and that was all. I also kept my long-standing appointment to be photographed by Chuck Close for *Harper's Bazaar*. Having your photograph taken by Chuck Close is like having an X-ray. There is nothing between you and him, no filter, no makeup, no flattering lights, and practically no space because he takes his photos close up and head on. "How am I going to do this?" I thought at first, then surrendered, "I'm just going to." The result was raw, very raw: My recovering face looked droopy and was laced with black smudges. I should have really hated the photo, but I kind of liked it because it was real. So did *Harper's Bazaar*, which ran it as a full page and it hung very large on one wall at the Pace Gallery in Beijing, and even more prominently at my exhibition in Los Angeles in 2014.

The Chuck Close shoot wasn't the last that made me hesitate. The hardest thing for me now is to be photographed; I've never really liked it, but at my age, it's twice as hard. Two shoots I've done recently with Terry Richardson have taught me a lot about the nature of beauty. I've known Terry since he was a toddler, when I was working for the photo agent Albert Koski, who represented his father, Bob Richardson. The first time Terry photographed me was for *Purple*, Olivier Zahm's very edgy fashion magazine. Olivier called me and asked if I would be the model for the collections in their spring/summer 2009 issue. "Are you insane? I'm sixty-two years old!" I told him. But he was so persistent that finally I laughed and told him, "OK, I'll do it, but only if you put me on the cover." "I can't promise you that," Olivier told me, "but I will try." Their last cover model had been Kate Moss.

The day of the shoot arrived, and the last thing I wanted to do was have my picture taken. My eyes were swollen. I was tired. I was supposed to model half the collections, and a young, professional model would do the other half. I desperately wanted to back out, but there was no way. After hours of dreading, I said to myself. "I will just do this as fast as possible." I couldn't let them see how unhappy I was, so I affected confidence, and exaggerated all of my movements. With Terry, it's quite easy to do that—he likes exaggerated movement. So I laughed, I was silly, and threw my arms out triumphantly. I ended up on the cover of *Purple* magazine at the age of sixty-two in only my stockings, my bodysuit, and a Maison Martin Margiela jacket made of blond hair.

For the fortieth anniversary of the wrap dress, *Harper's Bazaar* asked if I would be photographed by Terry again, this time as "the original wrapper" with the famous American rap star Wale. It was a wild idea and my team was enthusiastic about it, so I reluctantly agreed. When the day arrived, once again I woke up looking exhausted. It was a Friday, and it had been a busy week; I'd met with the mayor at seven a.m. on Monday, and it had been nonstop after that with design and merchandising meetings, interviews and speeches. Barry and I had had a dinner or a gala every night. I wanted to be alone in my car, driving to Cloudwalk, not in front of a camera, surrounded by young makeup artists and photographer's assistants, all staring at my tired face. But I put on the wrap dress they had chosen for me and told Terry, "Let's do it." Again I laughed, I posed, I exaggerated. And in the end, I loved the photo of me with my hand on my hip and my leg on Wale's knee. You can't tell my face is swollen when it's lifted by a huge smile. Clearly confidence is everything.

Confidence makes us beautiful, and it comes from accepting yourself. The moment you accept yourself, it makes everything better. I saw this in Nona Summers, who has been one of my best friends since we met at university in Geneva. Nona is this wild, glamorous, redheaded woman who was the inspiration for *Absolutely Fabulous*. She had been wild all her life . . . until the day she was diagnosed with retinitis pigmentosa, which meant she will eventually go blind. We were all very shocked at the news, but Nona took complete charge at the very moment she could have surrendered. That day she decided to get sober. To accept yourself, to be true to who you are, is the only solution to being fulfilled.

Zakia is another strong illustration of self-acceptance and its power. I met her at the 2012 *Glamour* Women of the Year Awards at Carnegie Hall when I was asked to give an award to Pakistani filmmaker Sharmeen Obaid-Chinoy for her Oscar-wining documentary on Zakia, an acid attack survivor. Zakia was asked to join us onstage, and her strength and quiet confidence moved the entire audience. After we left the stage, the three of us went downstairs to do some interviews. When I step into an elevator, I always check my makeup and adjust my hair, but in respect for what had happened to Zakia's face, I turned my back to the mirror. To my surprise, when Zakia stepped into the elevator, she faced it, gazing at her scarred image. I was awed watching her looking at herself, and embracing her image. Two operations and a skillful makeup job helped, but it was her dignity that made her very beautiful.

I certainly don't like to see my face aging in photographs, but I know if I wait ten years I will love those pictures. So I accept my image as who I am. What I found amusing about my ski accident was the number of people who said, "What a great opportunity for you to have a face-lift." Some did think I had had a face-lift and was just faking a ski accident. The truth is, I've never wished for my old face more than I did in the month or so following the accident. I didn't want surgery. I didn't want a new face. I wanted my old face back.

I know that people look at me and wonder why I have not succumbed to the progress of technology. Why have I not frozen or filled in the lines of my forehead. Why I have not clipped the bits of surplus skin on my eyelids. I am not sure, but probably because I am afraid of freezing time, of not recognizing myself in the mirror, the image I have been so friendly with. Losing the complicity with myself is something I would not like to happen, the wink in the bathroom mirror as I pass it in the middle of the night, the straight-on look that I recognize. My image is who I am and even if I don't always love it, I am intrigued by it and I find the changes interesting. I don't like the freckles and age spots that I have all over, but they are there, so I joke and say I have a printed skin like one of my favorite leopard-printed dresses. Even staring at the small wrinkles that curl around my lips can be interesting. They just appear one day at a time.

In my older face, I see my life. Every wrinkle, every smile line, every age spot. My life is written on my face. There is a saying that with age, you look outside what you are inside. If you are someone who never smiles your face gets saggy. If you're a person who smiles a lot, you will have more smile lines. Your wrinkles reflect the roads you have taken; they form the map of your life. My face reflects the wind and sun and rain and dust from the trips I've taken. My curiosity and love of life have filled me with colors and experiences and I wear them all with gratitude and pride. My face carries all my memories. Why would I erase them?

I don't judge those who choose to have cosmetic procedures. I sometimes contemplate the idea, ask around, get a phone number of a doctor, and then forget. I may one day, out of the blue, decide to do something myself, but until now I have chosen not to. I cannot pretend that I am younger than I am, and truly I feel that I have lived so fully that I should be twice my age. It is no longer about looking beautiful, but about feeling beautiful and fulfilled.

The other day I was struck by a bouquet of garden roses that was on my night table near my bed in Paris. There was one particularly lovely rose in this fragrant bouquet. Days went by, and slowly the rose began to fade. Even fading, it maintained its beauty. Some of the petals dried, curled, and had little brown spots on them, giving it a special beauty that was different from the beauty it had when it was fresh and new. I felt connected to that rose. Every time I see a new imperfection appear on my face, I think of that rose and how beautiful it was. I want to grow to be that rose.

Because of my work, I'm fortunate to be surrounded by youth and beauty—the models, the young women who work in my studio. They are a tonic for me. They make me feel young.

My surroundings are beautiful, too, which is very important to me. The six-story DVF headquarters at 440 West Fourteenth Street in the old Meatpacking District is filled with light. The building is a model of "green" technology, of which I am very proud. It has three geothermal wells that heat and cool it. The interior is lit by a "stairdelier," a broad light shaft of a stairwell that runs all the way up from the ground floor to the "diamond" prism glass penthouse on the roof, where I sleep when in New York. There are mirrors and crystals along the central stairs to direct the natural light into all the interior spaces. The garden outside my glass aerie on the roof is planted with wild grasses, which, even though it's in a working environment in a busy neighborhood, makes it an oasis of beauty and peace.

I love sleeping on the roof. My glass bedroom feels like a tree house, a comfortable urban tree house. I look out at the New York skyline and the Empire State Building from my bed, which is nestled under a tent of linen panels. The freestanding bathtub is teak, reminding me of Bali. When I was a young mother, I lived in an old, established building on Fifth Avenue and felt very grown up. Now a grandmother, I live like a bohemian and it keeps me feeling youthful. When in New York during the week, Barry and I sleep apart, he, uptown in his apartment in the Carlyle hotel, I on Fourteenth Street. I like our arrangement; it makes our weekends and vacations all the more special.

No place, however, is more beautiful than my home, Cloudwalk. However blessed I am with energy, I need quiet to preserve it. I find it in the beauty there—the apple orchards, the openness of the green lawns, the Balinese flags along the river, the basso profundo song of the frogs. I was fortunate to have bought what was then a fifty-eight-acre farm for $210,000 when I was only twenty-seven. I'd fallen in love with it without even getting out of the car and immediately handed the startled real estate agent a deposit check. I have spent every possible minute there ever since. The trees at Cloudwalk have been my friends for forty years. I'm sure if I were sawed in half, our rings would match.

Nothing makes me feel more thankful than Cloudwalk. Nothing is more peaceful and reassuring. My children, Barry's love, Cloudwalk, and my work have been the most consistent things in my life. All my memories, all my photos, letters, diaries, all my archives are stored there.

I can spend hours sitting in front of the fourteen-foot-long desk created by George Nakashima out of a single piece of wood, reading and working. Barry and I like to read and be silent. Our dogs are by us, Shannon, the old Jack Russell terrier that Barry found on a bicycle trip in Ireland; Evita, a new Jack Russell puppy; and two terriers we brought home from a recent trip to Chilean Patagonia.

But what brings me to Cloudwalk more is the beauty of nature. The older I get, the more important it is to me. The fact that we cannot control nature appeases me and somehow brings me back to a normal dimension. Whereas my size is magnified in the city where everything is man-made and every problem is mine to be fixed, when I go on a walk in the forest and climb the hills around Cloudwalk, I feel small and I like it.

Nature is never still. Things are growing, ripening, aging, fading, and then starting again. The trees are beautiful even when bare. I love every phase and I am endlessly fascinated by that life cycle moving on. Nature never stops. Sometimes it can be cruel, bringing droughts or floods. Sometimes it's scary, spawning tornadoes and hurricanes. It can be unpredictable. We were hit one recent autumn by an early snowstorm that killed many trees and left us without power for weeks. I was sad to lose those trees that have been my companions, but I think it's good to be reminded of how little we are, how vulnerable.

One of my favorite walks at Cloudwalk is through the white pine forest to a sunny open field, then on to the side of the hill where I've chosen to be buried. For years, every Saturday I would go on a walk around Cloudwalk trying to think where I wanted to be buried. First I thought it would be in the woods among the beautiful stand of cathedral white pines, but then a few years ago the farm next door was put up for sale and to save the eighty-six acres from being turned into a housing development, we bought it. My original choice suddenly seemed too close to the house, so we chose this new spot as a meditation garden and a future burial place. I asked my friend Louis Benech, the French landscape architect, to think about it and he did a beautiful, simple design of two half-circle walls set in the hill. Victor, who, with his wife, Lourdes, has cared impeccably for Cloudwalk for years, has now built those walls with local stones. It is a special, quiet spot. Visitors to Cloudwalk always make fun of me for taking them to visit my future burial ground, so for now, we call it the meditation garden.

I love Cloudwalk and its beauty. I love to watch the sun set from one of the little stone walls and look out at the gorgeous views. I feel I become that view, that blend of meadow, forest, and hills. I am privileged to have all this beauty in my life. I worked hard for it and I'm still working hard. It's satisfying to know that one day, as far away as possible, this perfect land will be the place of rest for the woman I set out to be fifty-seven years ago in Brussels at Mireille's tenth birthday party.

THE
BUSINESS
OF FASHION

I didn't dare call myself a designer for many years despite the over-whelming success of my wrap dress. Yves Saint Laurent was a designer. Madame Grès was a designer. Halston was a designer. Me, I came into fashion almost by accident in the hope of becoming financially independent. I never dreamed that the simple dress I launched in 1974, a dress that was easy, sexy, elegant, and affordable all at the same time, would catapult me into fashion history. Yes, I'd sold millions of dresses by 1978. That dress had been inducted into both the Metropolitan Museum of Art's Costume Institute and the Smithsonian Institution collection, though I'm embarrassed to say I didn't even know what the Smithsonian was at the time. At the age of twenty-nine I'd even made the cover of *Newsweek*, which identified me as "Dress Designer Diane von Furstenberg."

Still, I didn't dare call myself a designer then, any more than I dared call myself a good mother while my children were still growing. You cannot make these claims until you get much older, because you need to have the proof, and so it wasn't until after I discovered I did have a second act, that I could do it again and be relevant and be right that the first time was confirmed, that it wasn't an accident. Only after almost two decades since I'd created the wrap dress, did I call myself a designer.

Looking back, what has been a whirlwind life in fashion fits neatly into three distinct phases: The American Dream, The Comeback Kid, and now, The New Era. This third phase, which I'm just moving into now, promises to be the most fulfilling. The goal is ambitious: to capitalize on all that I have done before and create a legacy for the brand so it will last long beyond me. The process has been painful at times and stressful, but the result, I hope, will be worth it. For me, it already is. To still feel relevant and so engaged at my age is a wonderful adventure. In a lot of ways, I am doing the same thing I did the first time. But finally I can use my experience and my knowledge to form a long-term vision. My instinct remains the constant. Being impulsive is my most valuable quality, though it is also my biggest fault. I have to caution myself, but it is still the driving force behind the brand, and amazingly, forty years after its birth, the wrap dress and I are still here and kicking.

I owe everything to that little dress: my independence, Cloudwalk, my children's education, the trips we took, the donations I make, the Bentley I drive, my place in fashion history—it all comes from that one little dress. That one little dress has taught me everything I know about fashion, women, life, and confidence.

I did not think much of the little wrap dress when I created it, but I now appreciate its value and uniqueness.

Looking back, I can't help but think, what if? What if I'd never met Egon? Gotten pregnant? Felt driven to support myself after we married? What if I hadn't met Angelo Ferretti in Cortina or Diana Vreeland in New York or Halston or Giorgio Sant'Angelo? What if?

I've long believed that the "ifs" were the doors to my future, and I dared to open them, one by one, as they came along. I knew the kind of woman I wanted to be but I didn't know how I would become her. Opening those doors led me on a path to fashion, and that became the path to the woman I am today.

4

THE AMERICAN
DREAM

The journey began after Egon and I left Geneva in 1968, he to New York to train at the Chase Manhattan Bank, I to Paris to look for a job. We were both twenty, too young to think seriously about a future together, so we each set off on our own adventures. It was in Paris that I discovered a world I didn't know, the glamorous world of fashion, which would seduce me forever.

I stumbled into it through my best friend in Paris, Florence Grinda. Florence was a vivacious socialite whom I'd met in Geneva but became close to at a party in St. Tropez. Her husband, the tennis champion and playboy Jean-Noël Grinda, had disappeared into the bushes with a Swedish model when I found her sitting alone and feeling sorry for herself. We started to talk, and to console her, I took her to the port for an ice cream. We became best friends, and when we returned to Paris, night after night I left my tiny ground-floor studio on avenue Georges Mandel in the 16th Arrondissement to go out with Florence and her husband. Through her I met exciting people and got invited to lots of parties. She got designers to lend me clothes, a common practice that was new to me. A fun new world was opening. However, what I desperately wanted was a job.

A friend of hers introduced me to the handsome and mysterious fashion photography agent Albert Koski, who represented all the best fashion photographers of the time: David Bailey, Bob Richardson, Art Kane, and Jean-Louis Sieff, among others. Koski hired me on the spot to be his assistant, his do-everything girl, from answering the phone in the little house in which he worked and lived in the 16th Arrondissement to curating the photographers' books to send to advertising agencies and magazines. That house on rue Dufrenoy was a beehive of talent filled with cool photographers and young models, a hot spot of glamour, beauty, and fashion.

I was much younger and certainly greener than all the people coming in and out of the office and was a bit intimidated by it all, though I was determined not to show it. It was my first involvement with models, many of whom came to rue Dufrenoy. The big models were Jean Shrimpton and Veruschka, probably the most beautiful women ever; Twiggy and Penelope Tree, the strangest ones; and, of course, Marisa Berenson who, along with Florence, was to become my best friend and godmother of my son, Alexandre. From Italy, there were Isa Stoppi, Albertina Tiburzi, Marina Schiano, and Elsa Peretti, who became the successful jewelry designer for Tiffany. There were also Americans, Cheryl Tiegs and Wallis, along with the timeless, forever magical Lauren Hutton. I did not meet every one of them then, but I dealt with their photographs all day. They were all Diana Vreeland's "girls." As editor in chief of American *Vogue,* she had invented them.

Working for Albert Koski was an invaluable indoctrination, though I didn't see it at the time. I was assimilating a lot of information without totally comprehending it, but assimilating it nonetheless. In years to come, I would often refer back to what I learned there. It's only in retrospect that you realize that all the little experiences add up to a whole. What I did know then was that the world of fashion was fun, glamorous, very cool and I loved it. It was 1968. Everyone felt free, acted laidback, and projected an image of being bored, though we were anything but.

It was then that I realized that fashion was a huge industry, a long chain of professions linked together. It started from the fabric mills making fabrics to designers making clothes and models showing them. Editors would choose them, photographers and illustrators and writers captured them, and magazines printed them. That long chain of inspiration, talent, emotion, and ideas would end with the women buying and enjoying fashion.

I became aware of trends, the must-haves of the moment. Big, clunky costume jewelry was in, fueled by the antielitism era of counterculture youth. So were big belts and hippie clothes—Indian silks, Afghan embroidered coats—and long hair, furs, and jewelry for girls and boys. Hairpieces, fake eyelashes, hot pants, and platform shoes were in and I wore them all.

Marisa Berenson was the perfect "it" girl of the time. She had traveled to meet Maharishi in India with the Beatles and was on the cover of *Vogue* covered with bold turquoises and corals. She was the image of glamour. I met Marisa through Florence and we immediately became friends. We were barely twenty but Marisa was already a top model. She was tall, skinny, and very elegant, and, like a chameleon, could transform herself into many different creatures of beauty. I saw a lot of her then. On the weekends, we would do a marathon of movies, going from one movie theater to another, crying watching Vanessa

Redgrave in the tragic role of dancer Isadora Duncan and laughing at the Stanley Donen comedy *Bedazzled*. We would end up late at night at La Coupole in Montparnasse to eat oysters, meet friends, and go on to nightclubs.

Marisa lived with her grandmother, fashion designer Elsa Schiaparelli. At the time Schiap (as people called her) was no longer working. She was an old, ailing lady, retired in her *hôtel particulier*, a grand townhouse on rue de Berry. Although her terrifying presence could be felt throughout the corridors, I never met her. Marisa, who would go on to become an actress, working for director Luchino Visconti in *Death in Venice*, Stanley Kubrick in *Barry Lyndon*, and sharing the screen with Liza Minnelli in *Cabaret*, had her own side entrance through the garden.

I remember being at that house with Marisa one day when she received an invitation to go to Capri to a fashion weekend called "Mare Moda." She asked me to go with her, but I didn't have the money. When I told her, she plunged into her handbag and gave me a few five-hundred French franc notes to buy my ticket. I will never forget that generosity, nor will I forget that very glamorous fashion weekend on the Mediterranean island. We dressed up eccentrically, stayed out late, laughed a lot, and flirted with attractive young Italian playboys. Marisa was a top model, but, to my surprise, I managed to hold my own.

That weekend turned out to be more than just fun. It was there that I ran into Angelo Ferretti, the flamboyant industrial fashion tycoon whom I had met once before at Egon's house in Cortina with his lovely wife, Lena, and son, Mimmo, the best friend of Egon's younger brother, Sebastian. Ferretti and I had become friends in Cortina, and we were happy to meet again in Capri. After I told him about my work with Koski in Paris, he invited me to come to Como, visit his factories,

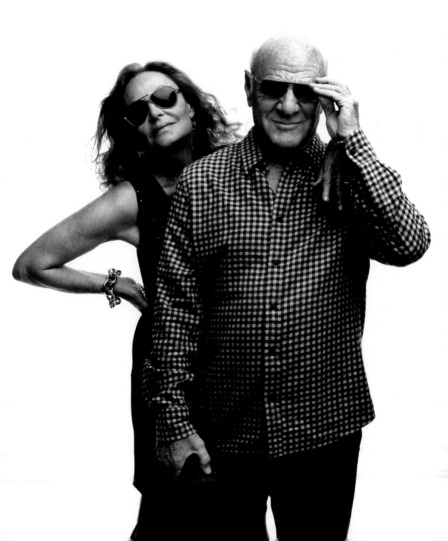

With Barry in Sun Valley, 2013. *(Jonas Fredwall Karlsson)*

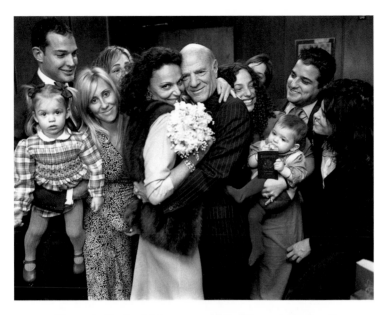

Surrounded by the children, my wedding to Barry, on the day of his birthday, February 2, 2001. *(Annie Leibovitz, courtesy of the artist)*

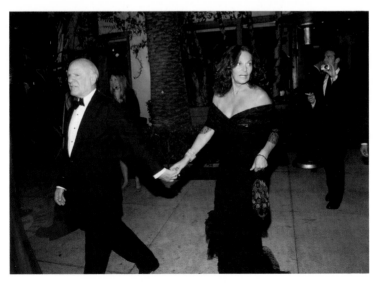

With Barry at the New York Public Library gala in 2007.

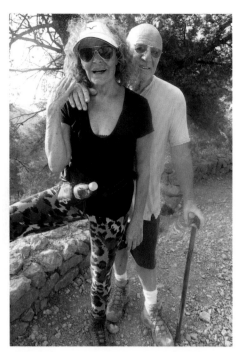

Hiking with Barry.

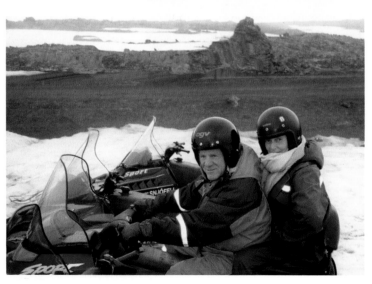

In the glaciers of Iceland with Barry.

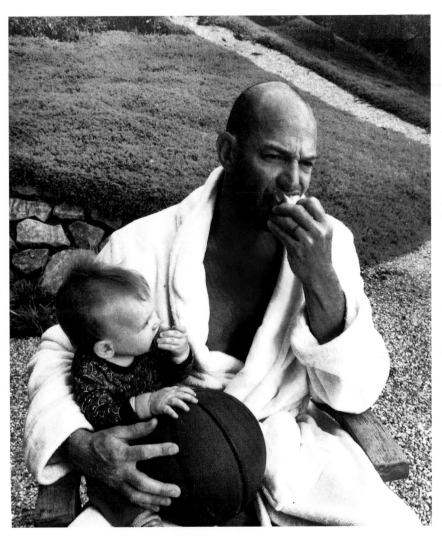

Alexandre with his son Leon, eating peaches.

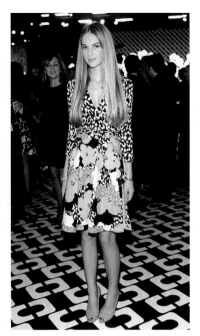

My granddaughter
Talita in a Warhol
wrap at the opening
of *Journey of a Dress*.
(Courtesy of Getty Images)

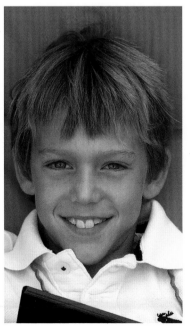

My grandson Tassilo.

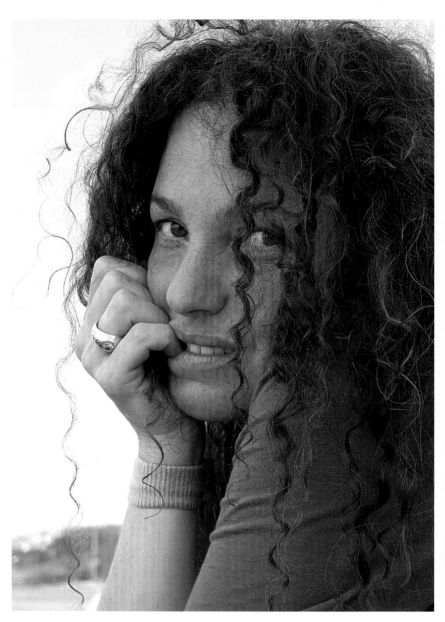

Tatiana in full beauty, captured by me, 2011.

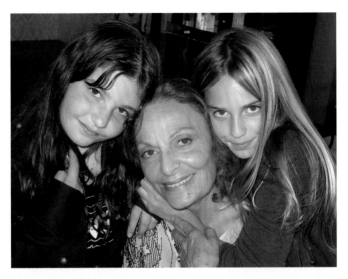

With both my granddaughters, Antonia and Talita.

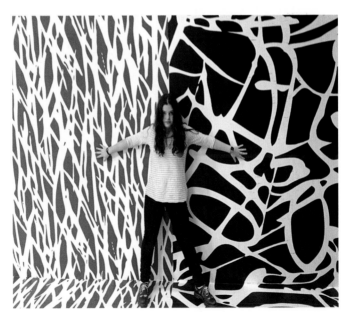

Antonia, Tatiana's daughter.

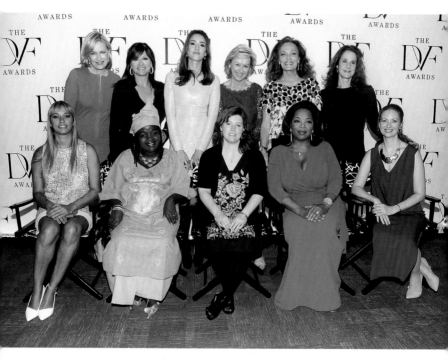

DVF Awards 2012 honorees and presenters. *(BFA Image)*

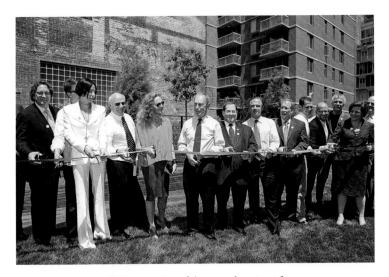

Ribbon-cutting of the second section of
the High Line, 2011. *(Joan Garvin, courtesy of the artist)*

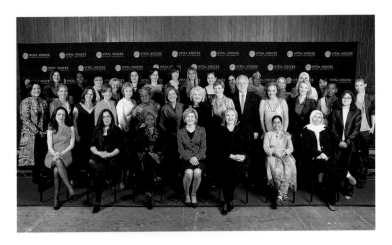

Vital Voices awards ceremony, 2011. *(Joshua Cogan, courtesy of the artist)*

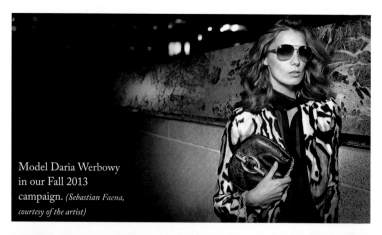

Model Daria Werbowy in our Fall 2013 campaign. *(Sebastian Faena, courtesy of the artist)*

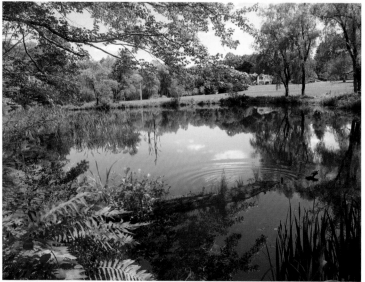

Cloudwalk Farm.

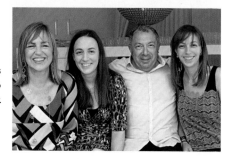

My brother, Philippe, his wife, Greta, and their two daughters, Sarah and Kelly.

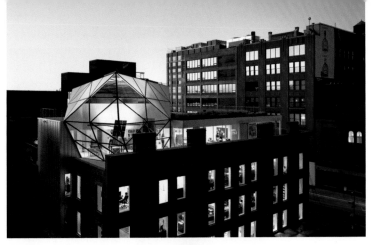

DVF Headquarters. *(Elizabeth Felicella, courtesy of Work AC)*

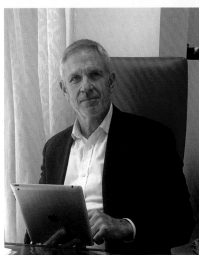

Joel Horowitz,
DVF cochairman.
(Michael Horowitz)

Spectacular Red Ball at Zhang Huan's studio in Shanghai, 2011.

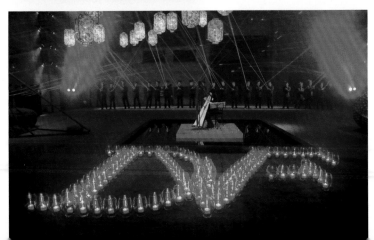

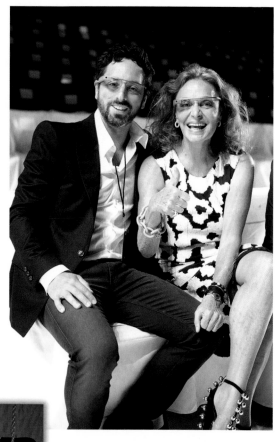

With Google cofounder Sergey Brin showing Google Glass for the first time. *(Greg Kessler, courtesy of Kessler Studio)*

Upside-down doing yoga, and on the phone.

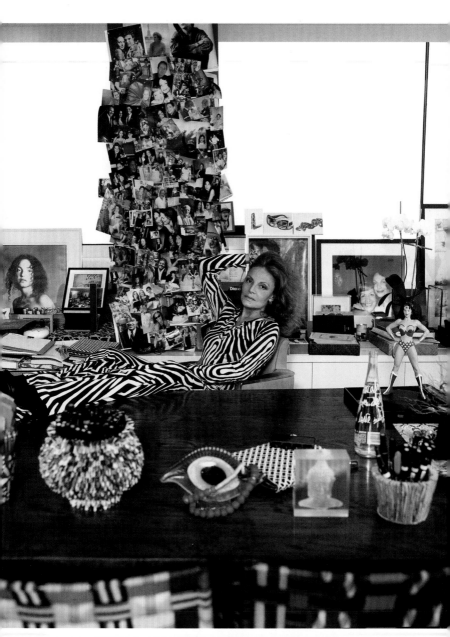
At my desk, surrounded by photos of my loved ones. *(Thomas Whiteside)*

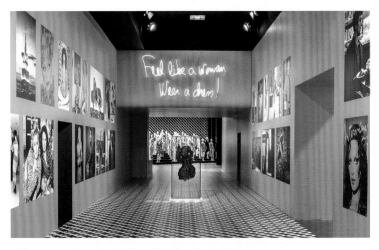

Entrance to *Journey of a Dress,* Los Angeles, 2014. *(Fredrik Nilsen, courtesy of the artist)*

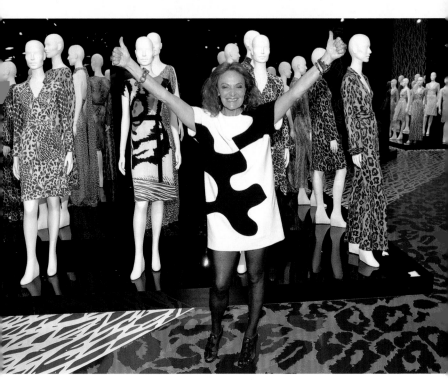

Moment of joy at the press conference for *Journey of a Dress. (Courtesy of Getty Images)*

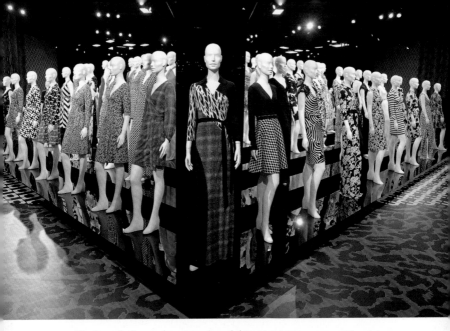

The "army" of wrap dresses at the exhibit. *(Fredrik Nilsen, courtesy of the artist)*

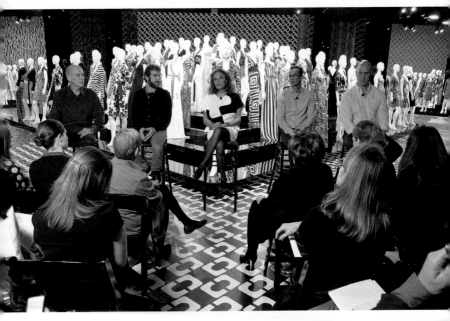

Press conference at the opening of the *Journey of a Dress*
exhibit on January 10, 2014. *(Courtesy of Getty Images)*

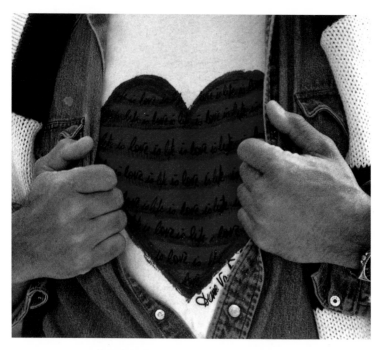

My first "Love is life" on a 1991 postcard.

and learn about his business. It was an intriguing and unexpected offer. Ferretti was on the other side of fashion, the manufacturing side.

He owned two factories in Pare, near Como, Italy: one, a printing plant where he printed intricate colorful scarves for Ferragamo, Gucci, and other large companies; the other, next door, where he produced knitted silk and high-quality mercerized cotton jersey fabric for shirts and T-shirts. A T-shirt seems like the most common thing now, but it was a novelty at the time. Until then, T-shirts were worn as an undergarment, mostly by sailors. But fashion T-shirts became the hot new trend in the late sixties when Brigitte Bardot started to wear those sold at Choses, a boutique in the port of St. Tropez. They came in a variety of colors and had an anchor with the words "St. Tropez" printed around it.

Ferretti was a pioneer in mass-producing his own upscale T-shirts, having converted old World War II silk stocking knitting machines to knit contemporary jersey fabric since silk stockings had been replaced by nylon panty hose. He also came up with the idea of printing on the jersey and using it to make new, bolder T-shirts. He was a genius really. He was also very much an Italian man: handsome, a serious gambler, a bit of a flirt, and great fun.

Ferretti's invitation to learn from him was tempting. "I'll think about it," I told him. Truth was, for all the glamour of Paris, I wanted to go somewhere else. Paris was a mess. The students had gone on strike in the spring of '68 and occupied the Sorbonne, soon followed by the workers who went on a general strike and shut down the airports and train stations. I was the age of the demonstrating students and I sympathized with them, but I must confess that my time crossing the barricades was mostly going to and from Régine's New Jimmy's nightclub on boulevard Montparnasse.

That summer I left Koski and took Ferretti up on his offer, moving in with my mother at her new apartment on rue Pergolèse and commuting back and forth to Italy to watch Ferretti operate and learn from him. Many years later, Koski would come back into my life, as he fell in love with my dear friend the screenwriter and director Danièle Thompson. Every summer, they spend time with Barry and me on our boat.

I see myself as if it were yesterday, sitting behind Ferretti in his printing factory as he is yelling at the colorist who made the yellow too bright or the pink too pale. I see myself sitting behind him at his fabric-knitting factory and he is yelling, yelling, at the engineer who has knitted the jersey fabric too tight or too loose. Always screaming, always passionate about the quality of his printing or the tightness of his jerseys, while I sit behind him watching and learning.

Como was the Italian center of silk and attracted a huge community of illustrators and artists who sold their artwork to the silk manufacturers. Through Ferretti's eyes I learned how certain designs can make good prints, how to create a repeat, and the difference between printing in application on greige or in discharge on a dyed fabric. I learned from his talented colorists how to create a harmonious palette and from him how to negotiate the prices of the designs. I realize today what a supertalent Ferretti was and how lucky I was to sit in with him creating patterns and watching the plain fabric going from screen to screen to screen to become colorful, precise prints.

He also taught me everything about jersey. He showed me how to evaluate the quality and density of the knitted fabric samples when they were brought to him, presentations that usually prompted the most yelling of all. I sat in on passionate meetings with the fiber engineers.

Jersey, I learned, can be knitted with many fibers, usually silk, rayon, cotton, or acrylic. "Mix is the magic, just like in cooking," he used to tell me. He was also a great cook, and his favorite dish was *bollito misto*.

I learned about dyeing and finishing techniques, about using imbibing agents to give the fabric breathability, and why, with certain fibers, the fabric gives or doesn't give. I learned all this and more just by sitting behind him in all the meetings with these talented, skillful technicians who had learned from their families for generations. I thought I was doing nothing, but every single thing I heard, I ended up later putting to use.

Soon after I'd started shadowing him, he bought a new factory near Florence, which was making fine, slinky nightgowns. The factory had excellent equipment and the perfect needles to work on jersey fabrics, and he converted it to manufacture his shirts and T-shirts. From that moment, Manifattura Tessile Ferretti became a vertical operation from fibers to knitting jersey to printing to finished clothes. The conversion of the new factory prompted more yelling, but I'd gotten so used to it I hardly paid any attention. What I did take in was the development of an amazing manufacturing company that would soon have a huge impact on my life.

Many of the things I still do today, I learned from that man. I had no idea that would happen, which is something I always tell young people. "Listen, always listen. Most people at the beginnings of their lives don't know what they want to be unless you have a real vocation, like a pianist or a doctor, so it is very important to listen. Sometimes there are doors that will open and you think it is not an important door and yet it is—so it's very important to be curious and pay attention, because sometimes you learn and you don't even know you're learning."

I spent almost a year with Ferretti, and learned so much, even though I was distracted. I was thinking about Egon and my heart was heavy. I knew Egon was coming home to Europe for the winter holidays and was taking his new Italian girlfriend, not me, to his family's house in Cortina. He was stopping first in Paris and he asked me to arrange a dinner at Maxim's with our Geneva University friends. Although it was a painful evening, I didn't show it. I made a huge effort to be cool, smooth, and funny so Egon wouldn't know how fast my heart was beating as he stared at me from across the table. I was even more depressed because of the fortune-teller I'd been to that afternoon who told me I would be married within a year and traveling far away. What nonsense, I thought. I was in love with Egon and knew I'd lost him.

For all my unhappiness, I refused to mope. I had a life to live, after all, with or without him, so after spending Christmas with my father and Philippe skiing in Crans-sur-Sierre, I went to St. Moritz to join Marisa for the New Year. The Palace Hotel had a habit then, and probably still does, of giving a very special rate to young, pretty girls, and Marisa and I had a fabulous time, skiing, dancing, and laughing day and night. After the New Year, which was also my twenty-second birthday, who showed up but Egon. Without the girlfriend. It took only one night for our love to be rekindled, and with it, an invitation to visit him in New York. My mother gave me the best twenty-second birthday present ever—the airplane ticket—and the journey began toward that little wrap dress.

I stayed in New York only two months but that short time changed my life. I loved the city, I discovered. The people were alive, creative, and ambitious. There were no boundaries; everyone was young, doing interesting things and free of all the suffocating traditions and class distinctions of Europe.

I wanted to stay but I had to find some way to support myself.

Egon suggested I try modeling, which seemed a possibility after I met the famous photographer Francesco Scavullo at a party one night. "Let me photograph you," he said. I remember how nervous I was the next day as Way Bandy, the infamous makeup artist of the time, lined my eyes and added rows of false eyelashes while François, the French hairstylist, piled three hairpieces on my head. I posed topless, the very long hairpieces hiding my breasts. I was astonished with the result. "Could that seductive creature be me?" I wondered. With no hesitation I went to show the photos to the famous, grande dame model agent, the German-born Wilhelmina, expecting her to marvel and invite me to join her beauty stable. Wilhelmina looked quickly at the pictures while inspecting me from head to toe from the corners of her eyes. She was just as quick to coldly announce that I could never be a professional model. At least it was confirmed: Beauty was not what I should pursue as a career.

The busy social life I had with Egon in New York proved to be an important fashion education. Because I was Egon's girlfriend and he was so visible as a young, attractive aristocrat, various designers in New York, like those in Paris, offered me their clothes to wear. I spent time discovering the back rooms of those designers and saw how different the fashion in America was from Europe. In England it was the time of Carnaby Street, Biba, and Ossie Clark, influenced by India and the hippie movement. In France, fashion was more serious with couture and dressmakers leading the way, although in 1966, Yves Saint Laurent had cleverly democratized fashion by creating the first designer ready-to-wear at his Rive Gauche boutiques.

In America, fashion was different because of its large distribution through hundreds of department stores across the country. Seventh Avenue firms were running the show, keeping their designers anonymous. But a clever publicist, Eleanor Lambert, had the idea of bringing those designers out of the back rooms and into the spotlight. She created the Council of Fashion Designers of America and Bill Blass, Anne Klein, Geoffrey Beene, and Oscar de la Renta became celebrities. I fell in love with the new breed of designers—Giorgio Sant'Angelo, Stephen Burrows, Halston—who used soft fabrics, jersey, and bright colors. All that inspired me no end and as I left New York to return to Ferretti, I was excited, hoping I could learn more and one day create some things on my own to sell in New York.

I looked at all of Ferretti's resources with a different set of eyes when I went back to Como. He was extremely successful at making tens of thousands of silk scarves and jersey tops, but I believed more could be done with the incredible infrastructure he had built. The innovative uses of jersey I had seen in designs from Giorgio Sant'Angelo and Stephen Burrows inspired me, and an idea began to percolate in my mind. I wanted to try and make some dresses in the Ferretti printed fabric. I was drawn to the opportunity of filling the void I had seen in New York between the high-fashion hippie clothes and the stale, double-knit dresses. Maybe I could fill it with an offering of colorfully printed sexy easy jersey dresses.

I started to spend lots of time at the factory outside Florence and became friends with Bruna, the patternmaker. Together we made my first dresses: a T-shirt dress, a shirtdress, a long tented dress, and a long tunic with pants. We used whatever printed fabric was leftover in her sample room. Then, on my days in the Como factory, I spent hours going through Ferretti's archival prints, choosing some and begging Rita, Ferretti's right hand, to print some sample yardage for me.

The family had adopted me and I felt very much at home with them. Ferretti's son, Mimmo, was around a lot and he helped me, too.

We had fun working together. The Tuscan countryside around the factory was lovely and Mimmo and I used to have some great meals in the neighboring villages. Ferretti was encouraging and allowed me to carve out a small corner for myself in their sample room. Even though I was cautious, I knew it was disruptive. I now realize he must have seen in me some potential I didn't yet see in myself. He also introduced me to his tailor in Milan, and with him I started to drape some fancy evening clothes, but I was more comfortable in the factory working with Bruna on simple little dresses.

I don't know what my future would have been without the generosity and support of Ferretti. I was still working at the factory when I got pregnant and my life changed drastically. With my accelerated marriage to Egon, the dream I had of a career in fashion also accelerated. The only person that could help make that dream come true was Ferretti.

"This is what's happening," I said to him on a short trip to the factory in the midst of the wedding preparations. "I am pregnant, I'm getting married to Egon, and I'm moving to America. Please allow me to complete all the samples I have been working on and let me try to sell them in New York." Ferretti smiled and his response was more than I could have dreamed: "Go ahead. I believe in you and I think you will be successful."

I put a sample line together, most of it made with Bruna in Ferretti's printed jersey, except a few velvet dresses made by the tailor in Milan. All the clothes had easy shapes, were sexy in their simplicity, and packable for sure. One hundred dresses folded in a single bag. I was at another door to my would-be career. I could only hope it would open.

Egon and I married on a beautiful, sunny day, three weeks after his twenty-third birthday. I love the photo of us laughing and smiling under a shower of rice as we exited the town hall in Montfort-l'Amaury. It was taken by Berry Berenson, a young photographer and Marisa's sister, who later married actor Tony Perkins and was tragically killed on 9/11 aboard the first plane that crashed into the World Trade Center. That exuberant photo reminds me not only of our wedding day and of beautiful Berry, but right behind us, out of the five hundred guests, is Ferretti! There, in one happy image, are the two most important men in my life at the time, though I didn't know yet just how important Ferretti would be.

After a short honeymoon sailing the fjords of Norway and a great month with our friends at Liscia di Vacca on Sardinia's Costa Smeralda, I picked up my samples from the factory in Tuscany.

As I boarded the Italian liner *Raffaello,* I carried all of my hopes with me: the baby in my womb, and that suitcase filled with dresses. Egon had gone by plane weeks before but I insisted on sailing. I wanted to take the time to visualize my new life and arrive slowly in New York Harbor, past the Statue of Liberty, like any immigrant with an American dream. I had no idea how quickly that dream would come true.

When young people eager to start their own lives and careers ask me for advice I smile and always say: "Passion and persistence are what matter. Dreams are achievable and you can make your fantasy come true, but there are no shortcuts. Nothing happens without hard work."

That advice is the essence of my journey with the little dresses when I arrived in New York. Egon would go off in the morning to his new job at the Lazard Frères investment bank and, greatly pregnant and with my dream in place, I'd struggle out of the apartment with my suitcase full of clothes to make the rounds of department stores and centralized buying offices. The people I met were amused and intrigued by the unorthodox presentation of little jersey dresses pulled out of a Vuitton suitcase by a young, pregnant European princess, but it did not materialize into anything. I persevered, though, especially after the birth of Alexandre.

The door that opened two months later, in March 1970, was the most critical one in New York: that of Diana Vreeland, the intimidating, all-powerful dragon lady editor in chief of *Vogue*. It seems amazing to me now that I had the audacity to enter her fashion shrine and show her such simple little dresses. I had the advantage, of course, of having social status, but my youthful confidence is what made me push open that door. Diana Vreeland? Why not? And that was the beginning.

It was Diana Vreeland who first understood and appreciated the simple uniqueness of the jersey fabric and the easy, flattering fit of the dresses. They may have looked like nothing on hangers, but the dresses looked strikingly sexy and feminine when she put them on two of her in-house models, Pat Cleveland and Loulou de la Falaise, both of whom later became my friends. "How incredibly clever of you, and how modern this is," Mrs. Vreeland told me, ending our brief meeting with "Terrific, terrific, terrific." And along with my suitcase I was back out that door and facing another.

I opened that one, too, with the assistance of Kezia Keeble, one of Diana Vreeland's young and beautiful fashion editors. I had no idea what to do next as I folded my dresses back into the suitcase outside Mrs. Vreeland's office, so I asked Kezia. "Take a room at the Gotham Hotel on Fifth Avenue during fashion week. The California fashion companies show there. There will be a traffic flow of buyers around," she told me. "List yourself on the Fashion Calendar and put an announcement in *Women's Wear Daily*." I didn't hesitate. "Can I use your phone?" I asked as I sat at Kezia's desk.

I settled in a room at the Gotham Hotel and spent the first long days waiting for buyers. I had previously done some interviews and those early articles said much more about me being a socialite princess than the clothes I was showing, which, at first, I found frustrating. But that publicity prompted curiosity. Traffic picked up after several early articles in *Women's Wear Daily*, the *New York Post*, and the *New York Times*.

I was so excited to write the first order from a little boutique in New Jersey on my freshly printed custom order forms. Sales really began to gain traction the next season at the Gotham Hotel after my dresses appeared in *Vogue*. I remember large orders from Hutzler's, a department store in Baltimore, and Giorgio's, the fashionable boutique in Beverly Hills. Then Bloomingdale's came in. Their five-person team took over the room, discussing windows and advertising. I was overwhelmed. Not only was my English still a bit shaky; I understood nothing of the rag trade jargon.

T hose early years were difficult for many reasons. On one side Ferretti was not easy to deal with. My first orders of a few dozen dresses in a specific style was not what he had expected. "I have a factory, not a sample room," he insisted. Flying to Italy once a month, I would beg for his attention. He would yell. I would cry. "Stick with me," I kept pleading with him. When my orders were finally delivered they were often wrong—wrong color, wrong style, wrong size, wrong everything, yet whatever I shipped to the stores would sell immediately. That is what encouraged me to persevere.

I was totally on my own, with no experience, and the challenges were enormous. I remember Air India's freezing warehouse at Kennedy Airport, where, sitting on the floor sorting out a new shipment from Italy, I had to cross out all the labels written in Italian and rewrite them in English. I can see myself crying from the cold and exhaustion, but now, of course, that experience has become a fond memory. So has the way I stored the folded dresses in our dining room and shipped all the orders myself, while also handling the invoices.

My very first print was the chain link print, a black-and-white geometric design made in a button-down shirtdress that I wore sitting on a cube for the first announcement in *Women's Wear Daily* in 1970. In 2009, Michelle Obama, as the new First Lady, wore that same print I reissued in a slightly larger scale on a wrap dress for the Obamas' first official White House Christmas card. What a lovely surprise! Decades after I introduced the chain link print, it was still relevant, making it truly timeless. At the time I designed it, however, timeless had a different meaning. During those same first two years of my new business, I also had two babies. To say I was busy is a huge understatement.

It was really getting to be too much to do by myself. I could not keep running the business out of my apartment, so I took a tiny two-room office on West Fifty-Fifth Street that became a showroom, a warehouse, and an office all in one. Olivier, my best friend from Geneva who was now a photographer, would come in and help with buyers. I tried to convince some large Seventh Avenue houses to distribute the dresses. One after another turned me down. "These boutiquey little dresses could never sell in large enough volume" became the constant refrain. That door remained closed to me, but another far more important door opened when I met Johnny Pomerantz, the sympathetic son of one of those Seventh Avenue businessmen, who told me all I needed was a showroom on Seventh Avenue and a salesman.

I was twenty-five, in business alone in a new country, and totally inexperienced in the ways of the garment trade. "I don't know any salesmen," I told Johnny. "Call me in a few days," he replied. And so

Dick Conrad, a thirty-nine-year-old salesman with lots of experience who was searching for a new business to run, came into my life. He took a gamble and agreed to join me if I gave him $300 a week and 25 percent of my company. I could find the weekly amount and 25 percent of nothing is nothing, so we struck a deal. I put $750 into our new company, Dick put $250, and I signed a lease for a showroom on Seventh Avenue. We were in business!

I made a few men's shirts for Dick to wear in Ferretti's jersey so that he could experience and understand the uniqueness of the fabric. He did. Dick knew all the best buyers in the specialty stores and better department stores across the country and he called them all. They all came into our new showroom at 530 Seventh Avenue and bought. By the end of 1972, our wholesale revenues were $1.2 million.

Though Ferretti remained very difficult to work with, he generously financed us by allowing a long-term credit of 120 days so we had time to ship and get paid by our customers before paying him. Before we agreed to those terms, at one point we got so far behind I went to a pawnshop across the street from the New York Public Library and pawned the diamond ring Egon and my father had given me when Tatiana was born. (I bought it back four weeks later at enormous interest.)

First there was the simple, perfect T-shirt dress; my favorite, the shirtdress; and a very popular tent dress that came in long and short lengths. Then came a little wrap top, somewhat like the top ballerinas wear to practice, which I designed with a matching skirt. It sold out immediately. The ultimate breakthrough came when I saw Julie Nixon Eisenhower wearing the wrap top and skirt on TV speaking in defense of her father, President Richard Nixon, during the Watergate scandal. "Why not combine the top and the skirt into a dress?" I mused. And the concept for the wrap dress was born.

It wasn't easy to figure it out at first. I wanted to keep the wide belt of the top to keep the waist small, I wanted the skirt to be bias cut, the neckline low enough to be sexy but high enough to be proper, and I wanted a strong collar and cuffs, just like the original top. Bruna and I spent many hours at the factory outside Florence standing around the cutting table playing with paper patterns, figuring out the puzzle. Sue Feinberg, an Italian-trained American designer, worked with us, too. I'd hired her to oversee the production and design at Ferretti's factory. She and I used to spend half of our time naked, wrapping and unwrapping ourselves in dresses as they came off the table to check the fit. Finally, one did.

T/72—that was the number assigned to the first Diane von Furstenberg wrap dress produced in 1974. Forty years later, the dress is still alive. Wrap dresses had existed before, of course. A wrap is a very classical shape: a dress that closes itself without buttons or zippers, like a kimono. But this wrap was different because it was made of jersey. The fabric molded to the body in the most flattering way, and was incredibly soft and comfortable while at the same time tight enough to fit the body like a second skin.

The wrap dress made its debut in 1974 at a fashion show Egon and I, who had separated by this time, shared at the Pierre Hotel. (Egon had left the bank wanting to be a menswear designer and was showing a line of shirts he had designed also out of Ferretti's material.) For the wrap dresses I had chosen two animal prints: snakeskin and leopard. I wanted women to feel sexy, slinky, and feline in the dress and they obviously did. The wrap dresses and the animal prints took off like a stampede, and soon could be seen on the streets of cities all over America. Thanks to the little wrap dress, the business multiplied sevenfold.

Ferretti was very happy, of course; by the end of 1975, production had escalated to over fifteen thousand dresses per week. His factory near Florence was working for us in full capacity. Ferretti had believed in me and I had more than fulfilled his expectations. Over five years, I gave him $35 million in orders.

All of this without a business plan, without any market analysis, without a focus group, without a publicist, without an advertising or branding agency. What I did have was a very good idea, a talented manufacturer who was passionate about his product, and an ambitious salesman who believed in me and sent me all over the country to make personal appearances at different department stores. The stores loved promoting the arrival of a real, live, young princess who was designing easy, sexy dresses that most women could afford. I plunged into the fitting rooms to show the women how to tie the wrap and feel confident about their bodies and themselves.

But it went further. As I was watching women become more confident and beautiful thanks to these new dresses, I was personally becoming more and more confident and, therefore, feeling more beautiful myself. I was projecting what I was selling—ease and confidence. I was becoming one with the dresses and what they stood for. I did not know it then, but I had become a brand.

The pace of growth was dizzying. Suddenly I had close to a hundred people on the payroll, including the staff at the warehouse I'd had to rent on Tenth Avenue to house all the thousands of dresses arriving from Italy. That one little wrap dress had taken the world by storm and I was running behind it as fast as I could. Opportunities were coming in left and right, and as I was young, inexperienced, and not equipped to assess them all, I had very little way to discriminate and decide what offers to choose and for what purpose.

When various entrepreneurs started approaching me as early as 1973 to "license" my name and use my designs to put on their products, I didn't even know what that word meant. They were varied: a mom-and-pop silk scarf company, a Seventh Avenue veteran who wanted to sell shirts made out of Ferretti's fabric, a small luggage company owner who wanted to put my name on a new line of totes, a clever entrepreneur who decided to get into eyewear. I signed contract after contract until my name was on seventeen product categories. By the end of 1976, the licenses were worth more than $100 million in sales. I was twenty-nine.

Everything I touched seemed to turn to gold, including a cosmetics line I started with a friend simply because I loved cosmetics. The idea began to form after I lost all my makeup on one of my trips and went to replace it in an emergency, only to find that makeup lines in department stores looked and smelled old. They were very serious and not fun or relevant to the new, playful fashion mood. "If I dress women so successfully," I said to myself, "why could I not create colorful makeup they could play with that would make them even more beautiful?"

The makeup I was personally using and loved was the professional stage makeup sold at the Make-Up-Center a block from my first office. The little pots of reds, lavenders, turquoises, and purples were irresistible to me and I used to buy all the colors they had. I loved sitting on the big square sink in my bathroom with my feet in the basin to be close to the mirror and play with my face. I had a good face for makeup: lots of eyelid and strong cheekbones. I loved applying the makeup on others, too, and I got good at it.

The idea of turning that passion into a business was solidified in an unexpected way. I was in Los Angeles, staying at the Beverly Wilshire hotel. At the time I was having a mini fling with the movie star Ryan O'Neal. He had come to my room to pick me up for dinner and he teased me about the quantity of makeup I had in my bathroom. "Why do you need all this stuff?" he asked. He may have been a big movie star and I a starstruck young girl, but I could not let his condescension go unanswered. "I don't need it. I just like it," I replied. But when he persisted in patronizing me in that arrogant way, I came up with a boastful reaction. "I'm thinking of buying the company," I said. It was a bluff, of course, but right at that moment I decided to create my own makeup line and go into the beauty business.

It was a ridiculous caper, for sure. As much as I loved cosmetics, I knew nothing about the business. Neither did my friend Sylvie Chantecaille, who had just moved from Paris with her husband, Olivier, and a newborn baby, and was looking for something to do. Sylvie, too, loved cosmetics (she now has a very successful line of her own with her daughter, the grown-up baby Olivia, who I remember learning to walk amongst pots of makeup and creams), so we set out to learn what we needed to do, visiting laboratories and talking to experienced product developers. "You have to create a fragrance," we kept hearing. "That's where the money is."

I had no idea how to do that, so I hired someone who did, Bob Loeb, a beauty business consultant, and the three of us developed my first scent, a light, lovely fragrance named Tatiana after my four-year-old daughter. Tatiana's scent was a wonderful bouquet of white flowers . . . gardenia, honeysuckle, and jasmine. To introduce it, we sent out thousands of free samples by attaching a packet of the scent to the hangtag of the dresses I was shipping all over the country. Tatiana not only quickly became very popular when we officially launched it in

1975, but inspired a generation of new floral fragrances such as Revlon's Charlie, among others.

In the midst of perfecting Tatiana and developing a cosmetics line, I started researching and writing my first book: *Diane von Furstenberg's Book of Beauty: How to Become a More Attractive, Confident and Sensual Woman*. It was bold of me to feel I could dispense that advice at the age of twenty-eight, but wherever I went people wanted to know how I lived, what I ate, what I did for exercise, what makeup I wore. They wanted to know my secrets, so I decided to write the book. I didn't really think I had any secrets, but those questions made me think about the subject of beauty.

I had an ulterior motive as well. I wanted to learn all I could about the business of beauty. Researching for the book, I talked to many experts about nutrition, hair treatment, skin cleansing, exercise, cosmetics—everything to do with beauty. Evelyn Portrait, Bob Loeb's lovely wife, helped me with the research and the book did very well when it was published in 1976.

We officially launched our cosmetics line at the end of 1975 at a small salon I opened on Madison Avenue. I wanted women to have the same fun I did sitting on my bathroom sink and playing with makeup, so in my little store on Madison Avenue (real estate was cheap at the time), I installed four little bars and stools in the front room where women could experiment with testers. The boutique was my version of the Make-Up-Center, and I loved it. So did the women who came in unsure how best to use makeup, and left with lots of products and a personalized chart after a session with Nicholas, our professional makeup artist. Women wore a lot of makeup in the seventies, so our timing was just right.

I was happy with my tiny makeup venture—Sylvie and I did

it on a small budget, using stock packaging and working out of my apartment—and was a bit reticent to grow it beyond my shop on Madison Avenue. I was finally persuaded by the legendary Marvin Traub at Bloomingdale's to open my own cosmetics counter there and to go national. I was very involved with the dresses and my licenses and committing to Bloomingdale's would mean more salespeople, advertising costs, and a lot of my time, of which I had none. But I had fantasized about joining the ranks of such pioneers as Helena Rubinstein, Elizabeth Arden, and Estée Lauder, and did it anyway. It was a blast.

I went on the road with Gigi Williams, a makeup artist and hilarious travel companion, to promote the cosmetics and the dresses, as well as the publication of my beauty book. Gigi was hip and cute, a true downtown little girl with early piercings who was married to artist Ronnie Cutrone, Andy Warhol's favorite assistant. Gigi and I felt like rock stars touring the country, doing interviews at local news stations and visiting all the stores where long lines of women were patiently waiting for makeup applications. We loved doing those makeovers and making women feel more secure with a little eye shadow, a little highlight on the cheekbones, and, equally as important, a little pep talk (and of course a spray of Tatiana perfume).

More and more I was realizing from my conversations with women how many had insecurities. By listening to their insecurities and sharing my own, we all felt stronger. It was an authentic dialogue, a very even give and get. The stronger I became, the stronger I wanted others to be. I realize now that it was at that time, as I was feeling stronger, that my desire to empower women started, a desire that exists to this day, more and more.

Back then, however, my main goal was to be free and independent. I was constantly on the go. I loved being that woman high on her heels walking in and out of places like a tornado, taking planes as if they were buses, feeling pragmatic, engaged, and sexy. I loved the idea of being a young tycooness who smiles at her shadow and winks at herself in the mirror. I loved having a man's life in a woman's body. In a sense I had become the woman I wanted to be, and it was then, at twenty-eight, that I met Barry and we fell in love. He, too, was a young tycoon, barely thirty-three. We both were living an American Dream, separately and together.

My wrap dress had become the "it" dress and I had become a celebrity. I was identified with all my products and was the model for them, all that in no time at all. I had succeeded beyond my wildest dreams.

Even the staid *Wall Street Journal* took notice and on January 28, 1976, ran a feature about my "fashion empire" on the front page. I was beyond proud of myself that morning as I took a very early flight to Cleveland for a personal appearance (having young children, I tried to stay home with them at night and fly early in the morning). There were almost no women on that flight. I sat next to a businessman with my pile of magazines and newspapers on my lap. The *Wall Street Journal* was on top. After a few minutes of staring at me and my legs, huffing and puffing, trying to figure out how to start a conversation, the man asked, "What's a pretty girl like you doing reading the *Wall Street Journal*?"

I looked at him, but said nothing. I could have shown him my front-page story, but it seemed too easy, and to this day, the fact that I did not remains one of the best personal satisfactions I've ever had. I kept my triumph to myself. Though of course I have told that story so many times since that I have more than exploited this poor guy's chauvinist attitude, which was so common at the time.

Exposure attracts exposure and two months later, I was on the cover of *Newsweek*. That was a very big deal in those days before CNN and the Internet. President Gerald Ford had been slated for the cover, having just won the Republican presidential primary, his first since replacing Richard Nixon in the White House, but the editors must have thought I'd make a more appealing sell and decided to put me on the cover instead. When an urgent call came from *Newsweek*, I snatched one of my favorite green-and-white jersey shirtdresses off the rack and raced over to Scavullo's studio, where he squeezed me in for the photo in the midst of a cover shoot for *Cosmopolitan*.

The *Newsweek* cover ended any anonymity I might have had, which, at first, I found intimidating. I'd been invited to the White House just before the cover ran by Luis Estévez, the Cuban-born California designer who made First Lady Betty Ford's clothes. It was my first visit, so you can imagine my amazement to find myself seated at President Ford's table and joking with the president about *Newsweek* choosing me for the cover over him! It all seemed unbelievable, especially when Henry Kissinger introduced himself to me as if I wouldn't recognize him. He subsequently became a good friend and after he and his wife Nancy bought a home near me in Connecticut we often had dinner together.

We all know the value of publicity, but the *Newsweek* cover launched a tsunami. The story spiked sales of the dresses, with more stores fighting for them, and brought me a whole new and very profitable line of work: home design.

There is an energy and an audacity that comes with youth. Older people often find this unchecked spirit uninformed and irritating, and are surprised when that spirit triumphs. And so it was with me and Sears, Roebuck. I'd been approached shortly after the *Newsweek* cover by a bedspread manufacturer who wanted to put my name on the bedspreads he was making for Sears. Bedspreads? I thought. Why stop at bedspreads? At the time, Sears was a very powerful company with many stores and a large catalog on everyone's kitchen counter. They had enormous advertising power and would take out eight- to ten-page magazine ads showing an entire house. Why not give the Sears customers the choice of more interesting home products? Mine.

I put together some sketches and flew to Chicago to see the all-powerful Charles Moran, the head of Sears's huge home furnishing division, which did about $1 billion a year in sales. My mother often reminded me of that day when I left the apartment at six a.m. carrying a huge folder with my presentation. I think even she was impressed by my drive and energy.

I can see myself now in that boardroom with a lot of white, middle-aged midwestern men glancing at my sketches and staring at this strange creature from New York with masses of curly hair, a foreign accent, and a lot of leg trying to sell herself to design home furnishings for Middle America. I can only imagine what they were thinking when, in response to Moran's question of what I wanted in compensation for my work, I said I wouldn't do it for less than half a million dollars. That was an unheard-of amount in those days, but I was young and bold. As weeks passed I became afraid I'd pushed too far, but then I got the call that they had accepted my proposal. What I did not know was that when I signed the contract with Sears I broke a taboo. If you sold to upper-tier stores like Neiman Marcus and Saks you were not supposed to also sell to a mass merchant like Sears. But because my dresses were so hot in department stores, I managed to get away with it.

For the third time I set up a studio in my apartment and hired Marita, a young girl with great taste, to help me design what was in essence a private label line for Sears, The Diane von Furstenberg Style for Living Collection, which quickly grew beyond sheets and towels into curtains, tableware, rugs—eventually even furniture. It was a lot of hard work designing and color-coordinating the different products, then presenting them to the legions of Sears buyers in different categories, and I soon hired an experienced textile designer couple, Peter and Christine d'Ascoli, to manage the Sears collection. It was well worth it. In the seven years I worked with Sears, retail sales of my home furnishings line grew to $100 million a year.

No wonder I call this phase of my business The American Dream. Even I find it hard to believe, as I write this, what I achieved in so little time. In less than five years, I'd gone from a little European girl determined to support herself to achieving success that far exceeded that dream. I was only twenty-seven when I bought Cloudwalk, twenty-nine when I was on the cover of *Newsweek*, barely thirty when I bought a huge apartment on Fifth Avenue as a birthday present to myself.

There was a price for my success, of course. I always felt I had to run faster and faster just to keep up with the business, which filled me with anxiety. The anxiety proved to be justified when the American Dream turned into a nightmare.

I saw it coming, but my partner didn't listen to me. Neither did my lawyer, my accountant, or Ferretti, for that matter. I was the one on the road making personal appearances, noticing the racks and racks of printed jersey dresses in one department store and the racks and racks of the same dresses in the department store across the street. They, on the other hand, looked at the avalanche of orders after the *Newsweek* cover and supported the decision to up the production at Ferretti's factories, all wrap dresses: blue and white, red and white, green and white! Women all over the country had at least two, five, sometimes ten of those dresses, if not more, already hanging in their closets—and the market for them crashed.

I remember that Sunday in June 1977 when every department store in the city took a full page in the *New York Times* advertising the wrap dress on sale. I was so used to seeing the dress advertised that I wasn't particularly alarmed. I didn't realize the negative impact until the next day, a sunny Monday, when *Women's Wear Daily* announced that the market for my little dresses was "saturated," that the sales marked the "end of a trend." The dresses were still hot with the public, but overnight the market for new sales collapsed in department stores across the country. I was close to panic. Orders plummeted and I faced $4 million of dead inventory. What to do? The only thing I could think of was to immediately stop the twenty-five thousand new wrap dresses Ferretti was making each week. He was furious with me, but I had no choice. My company was on the verge of bankruptcy. I was in shock.

I felt even then, and know now for sure, that we had done it to ourselves. We had behaved like amateurs on a runaway horse. My instincts to diversify the offerings and expand from just making wrap dresses had been ignored when I reported seeing the glut on the market. That little dress was everywhere. I wanted to expand the dress into a collection, a wardrobe, but my associates didn't consider that the demand would ever end. I should have been more forceful in cutting back the orders after the *Newsweek* cover.

I separated with Dick Conrad, paying him $1 million for his 25 percent share of the company, hired a new president, replaced the lawyer and accountant who had ill advised me. I was now chairman, sole owner, and head designer of Diane von Furstenberg, Ltd. So it was I who received the letter from Roy Cohn, the most feared lawyer in America who had been Senator Joseph McCarthy's right hand. Ferretti had hired him to sue me. My heart stopped, but I didn't show my fear. I called Roy Cohn and screamed bluffs: "With all the things I know about Ferretti, I don't think you want to go after me," I threatened. Then I hung up. My bluff worked. I never heard from him again.

But I still had a huge inventory and an even bigger knot in my stomach. Barry was looking at my numbers and looking for a solution. He was incredibly supportive but knew nothing about the fashion business.

The good thing was that success had made me into a household name. The Seventh Avenue companies that had snubbed me a few years before were suddenly all interested in buying my business. It was another flamboyant fashion person who appeared in my life and saved me. I think of Carl Rosen as the "Seventh Avenue Ferretti": passionate and visionary. Carl had just made a deal with Calvin Klein to make a line of jeans. Now he wanted to sign a license with me to make Diane von Furstenberg dresses. Not only would he buy and dispose of my inventory, but he would run the business and pay me a royalty with a guaranteed minimum of $1 million a year. Barry negotiated the deal. Barry is known to be a tough negotiator but so was Carl. They went on for days. Only recently, Barry confessed to me that at one point he had pushed so far he thought he had blown it and that Carl would walk out. But he didn't.

Once again, my mother's credo proved true: What had seemed the worst, turned out to be good. I had managed not only to get rid of a terrible liability but also to work out a profitable arrangement.

My American Dream was still alive and well as I moved forward. Again, I drew on my mother. "If one door closes, another will open," she would say—and it did. My beauty line. It had done very well since I'd launched it in 1975, especially Tatiana, the fragrance, but with the dress business no longer my responsibility, I could now concentrate on taking the beauty line to new heights. Without a moment of nostalgia I got rid of my showroom in the garment district and moved uptown to glamorous offices on Fifty-Seventh Street and Fifth Avenue, in the heart of the cosmetics world. I leased the entire twenty-fourth floor in the old, art deco Squibb building at 745 Fifth Avenue with a view of Central Park and Revlon and Estée Lauder right across the street. I converted what the prior tenant had used as a storeroom into my private, airy, pink office with a terrace. I felt happy and on top of the world!

Since I was chairman and sole owner of the company, it was mine to make or break. I did not think much about funding the beauty business. All my licenses, including the dresses and my home furnishings for Sears, reached $150 million in sales and provided a large income.

My new president was Sheppard Zinovoy, and I hired a professional beauty salesman, Gary Savage, whom I lured from Pierre Cardin fragrance. A ravishing girl, Janet Chin, joined me as a product development person and I even built a state-of-the-art laboratory in the office that was run by an Italian chemist called Gianni Mosca. It all felt very serious when I put on a white coat to enter the lab and test the samples he and his assistant developed, and for me it was a dream come true.

Without the dress business I had the time to play with colors and textures and packaging design. In the seventies we all wore lots of very bright makeup and I had so much fun working with Janet creating and naming the colors and designing the packaging. At Gary's suggestion we named the line "The Color Authority," and indeed it was. I was proud, not annoyed, that other cosmetics companies, from Revlon to Estée Lauder, bought and copied our new colors the instant we released them. To me, anyway, imitation is the sincerest form of flattery. We redesigned the packaging. No more inexpensive stock packaging for us, but a lovely marbleized white plastic compact that looked like mother-of-pearl with my signature in gold. I've always said that makeup is the secret between women and their mirrors, and that makeup is a reflection of our moods. To that end we created compacts that incorporated all the colors you needed, divided into three different moods: Hot Passion Pinks, for a feminine, flirtatious mood; Stop Traffic Red, for strength and authority; and New Wave Metallics, for the browns of more neutral and quiet moods.

As the cosmetics line grew, so did the volume of different bottles, boxes, and caps, which we had to keep stored in a warehouse. It was déjà vu with the inventory of dresses, right down to the multitude of warehouse staff we needed to manage it all. Each product had its own packaging with its own list of ingredients. The many colors we had so much fun creating required their own labels with their own lists of ingredients. On and on. Overseeing and maintaining the line was very expensive.

For all that we loved working on the color line and the attention and success that greeted it, as we had been advised, it was Tatiana, in a new bottle custom designed by sculptor Serge Mansau, that was making the money and we expanded the fragrance into a whole line of bath products.

I also started to conceive of a new perfume. I wanted something very special with a strong scent, a unique bottle, and a passionate message. I called it Volcan d'Amour (Volcano of Love). Since it had been inspired by my Bali days with Paulo, I dedicated it to him.

I went all out with that fragrance, commissioning a magician-turned-designer friend, Dakota Jackson, to create a unique and expensive bottle, and commissioning another friend, Brazilian artist Antonio Peticov, to design the box it came in. Bloomingdale's and

Saks fought for the launch, which was an over-the-top event I staged in my office with pyramids of fresh frangipani I'd shipped from Hawaii to symbolize the offerings to the volcanoes of Bali. From the office we descended Fifth Avenue to Saks, where I dressed the models in blue sarongs I had designed and had had hand-painted with gold volcanoes at the Denpasar market.

What was I thinking? Yes, the company was doing very well. By 1981 we had gross sales of $40 million, but our expenses were enormous. The payroll for over three hundred employees was $1 million a month!

I began to feel tense about meeting that payroll and about the ever-growing inventory of bottles and tops and boxes. The sleepless nights I'd experienced from the panic of failure in 1977 were returning in 1982 because of the speed of our success. As the demand grew, I had to invest more and more money in inventory and a support system of staff and marketing. I was worried we were growing too rapidly again.

I know now, of course, that I should have read the huge, heavy financial reports that Gary Savage and Shep Zinovoy dutifully gave me every week, but I didn't. In my mind, they were in charge of the company's finances. I was the creative end of the operation.

Money, in fact, was the furthest thing from my mind as I explored the islands of Indonesia with Paolo to come up with promotional material for Volcan d'Amour. I trusted the men in New York to manage the money. I had no idea how overextended we were.

The end came as rapidly as that snowy January day when all my dresses suddenly went on sale. This time I was in Paris with Paolo when I got a call from Shep to tell me that I had to come back to sign a personal note of guarantee, and that Chemical Bank was refusing to lend any more money until I did. A personal note? That could mean the loss of Cloudwalk, the loss of my apartment. No way was I going to risk that.

The enormity of the crisis became clear when I got back. Ten million dollars!—that's how much the company owed the bank. I had no idea that we had been borrowing so much money to cover our operating expenses. I'd never read the financial printouts. The only way out was to sell the company. "If you can," the wretched little banker said.

It took months for me to negotiate a deal that could release me from the bank: a sale to Beecham, the big English pharmaceutical company that had started the process of accumulating small cosmetics companies to become a player in the industry. In New York, I felt the bank closing in as I poured my efforts and even more resources into the newly launched fragrance, Volcan d'Amour. But in London, I remember feeling so grown up in my suite at Claridge's hotel, talking with the chairman of Beecham about the future of my business.

To this day, Claridge's is my favorite hotel in the world and I was flattered when they asked me to redecorate a few suites for them in 2010 and make them sexy, luxurious, and glamorous. They were very happy with the result, and the suites have been booked solid ever since. When I see my photo hanging in their lobby, with Winston Churchill and Jackie Kennedy, I am immediately reminded how important I felt staying there, in spite of my panic over the looming debt back home.

The agreement I finally reached with Beecham was a great one. They raised their original offer to $22 million, plus royalties and a large annual consulting fee. I was ecstatic. The nasty banker got his money and I was still $12 million ahead. "Celebration," I wrote in my diary. "I feel free, rich and relieved." But I also felt sad. I'd sold something that really had spirit and was really strong. But I'd had no choice.

And so it was that the first phase of my business life—the American Dream—began to wind down. I'd accomplished more than I could ever have imagined and was extremely proud of the products I'd created. I'd built two companies and sold two companies. I'd more than achieved my goal of financial independence. I could retire, travel the world, and my children would always be secure.

On the one hand, it was liberating. I was thirty-six and for the first time in thirteen years I didn't have the pressure of running a company, and I was excited about that. On the other hand, I felt empty. What I realized later is that I had very little say in the design, quality, and most importantly distribution of the many licensed products. Little by little, the simple dress I'd made had disappeared. In the hands of Carl Rosen, his company Puritan, and the 1980s, the dresses were given shoulder pads and lost their identity as I had lost control. My name was on so many products, but I wasn't designing anymore; I had lost my creative outlet.

I missed that and realized how powerfully I missed it soon after the sale to Beecham when I went to A La Vieille Russie, a wonderful antique store in the Sherry-Netherland hotel, to buy myself a celebratory gift of jewelry. (I often buy jewelry to mark special moments. It signifies a commitment to myself—a ring, for example, when I break up with a man.) This time, while I was buying a beautiful set of aquamarine jewelry, I saw an empty shop for rent across the lobby. I decided to take it and, voilà. Briefly, at least, the American Dream was reignited.

My instincts told me that the elegant Sherry-Netherland on the corner of Fifty-Ninth Street and Fifth Avenue was a perfect location for a very upscale collection I could create for the extravagant eighties. The Carters had left the cloth-coat White House. The Reagans had moved in, complete with Mrs. Reagan's furs and designer clothes.

Millions of people were watching *Dynasty* and *Dallas* on television, and fashion and style changed enormously. The big hairdo and the big shoulder pads were in, as was Donald Trump and a lot of new money. It was not the New York I had fallen in love with, but I thought I could capitalize on the new extravagance and create something new of my own.

I commissioned the well-known architect Michael Graves to design what would be his first retail store. It seems crazy to me now that while he was converting the shop into a beautiful space I didn't even know what clothes I was going to put in it! Once again my impulsiveness had taken over. There wasn't a business plan at all, just a vision of creating couture-like clothes in exquisite fabrics. I thought an expensive, high-end line would strengthen the value of my name, and therefore help the other licensed products over which I had no control.

I hired a talented young Frenchman, Stephan Janson, to help me design this new line and Olivier Gelbsmann to manage the store. I called both the store and the new line by my first name only, Diane, and the first collection was exquisite. We used the most precious and expensive fabrics—silks from Italy, laces from France, cashmere from Scotland—and created elegant ball gowns and other eveningwear. I had lots of money from the Beecham sale, so I didn't need to skimp on anything, including the advertising introducing Diane in 1984. Image is all-important in couture. The clothes have to project high fashion, elegance, and be aspirational, so I hired Helmut Newton, the famous German photographer known for his strong erotic photographs, to shoot the campaign. I had always dreamt of being photographed by him and he loved the idea of using me as a model. We shot in an art deco mansion in the South of France and had a great time. They were beautiful images, which I treasure to this day—me in various Diane ball gowns and in my favorite, a black tuxedo with a veil over my eyes.

The early signs about Diane were very encouraging. An expensive ball gown of pink silk and black lace was bought over the phone and so were the rich tuxedos and evening pajamas. Brooke Shields, Bianca Jagger, and Ivana Trump were among my early enthusiastic customers. It all felt exciting.

The clothes were well made, beautiful, and absolutely right for the time, but looking back, I didn't really like that period in fashion. Nothing felt right. New York of the mideighties was not the same New York that had seduced me in the early seventies, and my personal life was also changing. My children had gone off to boarding schools and, emotionally, I needed something new.

Alain Elkann landed in my life at that very moment—an intelligent, attractive, needy artist in search of his own identity as a writer, as a man, and as a father to his three children. Rather than being excited about building yet another business, I was drawn to being Alain's muse and his partner in life.

I was drawn by the change in Europe, as well. There was the promise of a unified Europe that excited me. I bought lots of blue European Union flags with their twelve stars and displayed them all over my apartment. Newly elected French president François Mitterrand was an intellectual and the whole mood of Paris had become very seductive to me. I packed up, neglecting the fledgling business, and moved to Paris.

A little bit of New York came with me; my assistant, Ellen, who had been with me since she was nineteen, had just married a Frenchman and moved to Paris at the same time. Having each other made us feel a little less homesick.

And homesick I was. I never anticipated the huge identity crisis I would have, both personally and in my own sense of style. I had arrived in Paris with my beautiful newly designed clothes, but Alain didn't like them. That was when he bought me flat shoes and had me order tweed blazers from his tailor in Milan. A woman's style and what she wears reflects a lot of who she is, and I slowly became confused and insecure. I'd had my hair cut very, very short in frustration after the end of my relationship with Paulo, which required frequent visits to the hairdresser, something I'd not done for years. For the first time I began to feel older and started weekly facials. Even though I was in Paris, the epicenter of fashion, I turned my back on fashion and everything I had built. The new line and the Sherry-Netherland store in New York made no sense to me anymore. Soon after my move I closed it all down and sold my Fifth Avenue apartment.

I missed my children and wrote to them daily, while making myself a pleasant life in Paris. I spent my time with writers, and took great pleasure and pride in establishing Salvy, a small publishing company. That was a great plus during this very odd but instructive period in my life. I loved having a literary salon in my apartment and being a publisher, but as a woman I was learning who I didn't want to be.

5

THE COMEBACK KID

I wish I could say I quickly regained my confident, intuitive self when I left Paris in 1990 for New York, but it isn't true. I was quite lost. My business, what was left of it, was in tatters. The licenses had been sold and resold, and my designs had lost their point of view. My line of cosmetics had vanished in a series of mergers and acquisitions and the only survivor, the light, sexy fragrance I'd named after my daughter, was unrecognizable: Tatiana had been turned purple by its new owner, Revlon, and they had changed the scent.

Not only had I lost my brand, I felt I had lost my identity. I had not realized how much my sense of self had been linked to my work. I did not know who I was anymore. My children were both at Brown University and had blossomed into wonderful young adults. I was very proud of them. I was not proud of me.

What a fool I'd been. By altering my personality, I had now lost myself. By naïvely signing away my name on the licenses without any restrictions and by neglecting my business duties to satisfy my man, the brand had lost its character and much of its value. My income from the royalties had dropped by around 75 percent. When I visited some of the few remaining licensees in their offices, they paid little attention to my design suggestions or to me. In their eyes, I had become irrelevant. I was just someone who'd designed some hot dresses a while back and they couldn't wait for me to leave them alone.

At twenty-five, I was a wunderkind. At forty, I was a has-been. I started straightening my hair again. I hated what the licensees made so I could no longer wear the clothes that bore my name. After the easy jersey dresses, the sarongs of the Bali period, and the tweed jackets of my Paris life, my new personal uniform was couture jackets from YSL with tight Alaïa skirts or narrow Romeo Gigli pants. Trying to feel of the moment, I ordered lavish couture clothes from Christian Lacroix, the talented new French designer: dresses with big pouf skirts and embellished jackets. Those clothes were beautiful and relevant to the time, but not to me. I barely wore them.

I thought my insecurity showed on the outside, but evidently it didn't. Anh Duong, the artist who was modeling for Christian Lacroix at the time and later became a close friend, remembers seeing me for the first time at his haute couture house in Paris. "I was struck by how beautiful you were trying on Christian's clothes," she told me recently. I could not believe she said that. I remember feeling particularly desperate that day and far from beautiful. It proved to me once more that "the woman across the room" may appear perfect, yet does not always feel it. I certainly didn't. Though I spend so much time now telling young women to be their own best friends and that happiness is confidence, I was not practicing what I preached during that lost period of my professional life. I wasn't sure who I was.

I made a few false starts trying to get back to work. I signed yet another unfortunate license deal in 1990 to design a line of dresses, this time with a moderately priced company. The struggling company wanted to upgrade its image and was counting on my name to do it. The chairman had a beautiful smile and blue eyes and he convinced me with his enthusiasm. I went ahead because at least it would get me back into the stores. It did, for a very short time. The company declared bankruptcy the day the DVF division was to launch its second season. By then I had invested a lot of time in developing these new dresses and I quite liked them, so without thinking twice, I told the team I'd been working with at the licensee's office to move the dresses into my office and come work for me. Impulsive for sure, and short-lived. We delivered one more season but I was not equipped nor did I have the desire to rebuild a wholesale business.

"Forget the stores," I said to myself. "Why not go directly to my original, loyal customers who have not forgotten me?" On the wings of that idea, I flew to San Francisco with Barry to visit the powerful catalog house Williams-Sonoma. The catalog industry was booming and I was hoping that Williams-Sonoma would see the value of adding a Diane von Furstenberg catalog to their stable. We had a polite lunch with the chairman but the company was not interested in me, or any designer name. Barry and I left feeling defeated. Now we often laugh and share our fond memories of that day when we felt like two losers with our failed sales pitch.

Still obsessed with direct selling, I had an idea to create a magalog, half magazine, half catalog, and I asked the young graphic artist Fabien Baron to design it for me. He made a beautiful mock-up, but because I did not have the funds or the expertise to make it happen, the ridiculous idea remained on the shelf.

Something just had to happen, and something did, in the summer of 1991 in the Concorde lounge at JFK. I was on my way to join twenty-year-old Tatiana in Venice for a debutante ball given by Count

Giovanni Volpi in his palace. At the airport a man came rushing up to me. "Where have you disappeared to?" he asked me, and introduced himself as Joe Spellman, a marketing executive. "The world of fashion needs you again. You could be a major star of the new century." I looked at him incredulously but I sure enjoyed the recognition. Joe had been a marketing genius at Elizabeth Arden, and later Estée Lauder, and he was also consulting for retired Bloomingdale's chairman Marvin Traub. I met them several times when I returned from Venice. Joe came up with a startling idea: "How about selling on television?" he said.

I had never heard of TV shopping, but why not? Clearly it was a way to reach the customer directly. A few weeks later, on a Saturday morning, we all took the Metroliner train to Philadelphia. Then a car to the suburb of West Chester to visit a company called QVC. I had no idea what to expect when we walked into the live TV studio and saw soap opera star Susan Lucci selling hundreds of bottles of shampoos and hair conditioners in a matter of minutes, sales that raced on the computer up to $600,000! I knew in that moment that we had landed in the future, the world of teleshopping.

As I watched Susan talking directly to her customers through the television screens I became very excited. I envisioned myself reviving my cosmetics line on TV, but the QVC people had something else in mind. They wanted me to design dresses for them. I was hesitant, not really understanding how you could sell dresses on TV and, also, in fairness, a bit concerned about the "tackiness" of their presentation at the time. I told them I would have to think about it.

I reported my QVC visit to Barry. Coincidentally, he knew about the shopping network from discussions he had had with Comcast and Liberty, the cable companies that owned the station. The timing was fortuitous. Barry had left Fox and was also looking for a new direction.

Just as we had been two young, successful tycoons at the same very early age, at that moment we were both "unemployed" and looking for our next opportunities. Little did we know that both our next careers would start from the very same spot: QVC.

Back at my design studio, with the help of the young women I had inherited from the moderate dress company, Kathy and Colleen, we designed not dresses, but a concept we called Diane von Furstenberg Silk Assets. It was a line of washable, coordinated, printed silk separates and scarves. The styles were simple and did not need to be tried on: shirts with a generous cut; easy pants with elastic waists. The colors were bright and cheerful, the prints bold and pretty, and the pieces could mix and match in many combinations. Every mini-collection had an inspiration story. "Giverny" was the print story inspired by the palette of French Impressionist painter Claude Monet. "Pietra Dura" was another collection, inspired by Florentine marble. The stories created a narrative that was easy to discuss on air with enthusiasm.

Here I was, back to my roots, creating color palettes and designing prints. Equally exciting was the financial arrangement I made with QVC for them to buy the clothes directly from the manufacturer in Hong Kong. My responsibility would be to design the line, and make sure it was well made and arrived on time. I would then sell it personally on TV and do all the promotions. For that QVC would pay me 25 percent on top of their cost from the factory. It was a great deal for QVC and for the consumers because there was no intermediate wholesaler. It was an even better deal for me: I had no liability of inventory because the clothes would be shipped directly from the factory to QVC. That arrangement was a huge relief. After all, twice I had had to sell my company because I had not managed inventory properly!

The day I was to have my first Diane von Furstenberg Silk Assets show, in November 1992, I arrived in my hotel room at the Sheraton

Great Valley, next door to the TV studio, and found beautiful flowers with a note: "Welcome home and good luck! I love you, Barry." The "Welcome home" referred to Barry's secret and successful negotiations to take over control of QVC, launching him into the new world of interactive, a move he continued to build on to reach where he is today.

In two hours I sold $1.3 million of Silk Assets while Barry (who surprised me at the show) and the management of QVC watched the galloping sales figures on a computer. They were all cheering! Kate Betts, a young editor at *Vogue*, had come along to witness the first show and documented it with wonderment. "Show and Sell," her article began. "*Vogue* witnesses a fashion phenomenon in the making." Overnight, I went from a has-been to a pioneer once again.

It is not inappropriate to say that Barry and I put the teleshopping industry on the map. Barry's involvement in the new retail phenomenon legitimized it and my participation as a designer glamorized it. A steady stream of people started showing up in West Chester to witness the retail revolution. There were many, many stories about us and QVC in magazines and newspapers.

It just got better and better. Viewers couldn't get enough of Diane von Furstenberg Silk Assets. On one show in 1993, I sold twenty-two hundred pairs of silk pants in less than two minutes!

Success is not only glamorous, it's also a lot of work. Being on live television, often in the middle of the night, was exhausting, and driving back and forth on the New Jersey Turnpike made me feel like Willy Loman in *Death of a Salesman*. But the exhaustion was worth it; in very little time, Silk Assets generated $40 million in sales.

Barry sold his stake in QVC in 1996 and bought controlling interest in the Home Shopping Network. I followed him there with my business and sales continued to grow. The success of Diane von Furstenberg Silk Assets gave me confidence again, but on television

I could not sell the simple, body-hugging, more sophisticated dresses that were my own style. I missed that.

What I desperately wanted was to revitalize my signature brand and return to high-end stores. There were glimmers that it might just be possible. There was a growing nostalgia in the nineties for the fashion of the seventies, spearheaded by Tom Ford, who had revitalized Gucci and put the mood of that legendary decade back into motion.

"You should bring back your dresses," Ralph Lauren told me when I was pitching TV shopping to him, trying to persuade other designers to join me. Karl Lagerfeld and Gianni Versace said the same: "We love your original dresses. You should bring them back." Rose Marie Bravo, then president of Saks Fifth Avenue, agreed, asking me time and again to relaunch the little jersey dresses. Suddenly it occurred to me that I was some kind of icon of the seventies. In the new nostalgia, hip, young designers seemed excited to see me. I remember one day walking past Bar Pitti in the West Village where the edgy new grunge designers Marc Jacobs and Anna Sui were having dinner. They waved enthusiastically. I was surprised, to say the least, and very flattered that such hot young talents would notice me. Another young designer, Todd Oldham, named his fashion show "Homage to Diane von Furstenberg." Again, I was flattered though a little taken aback. "I'm not dead yet," I remember thinking.

The nostalgia for the seventies and my first designs kept growing. In New York, young girls, contemporaries of my cool daughter, Tatiana, were scouring vintage shops and thrift shops in pursuit of original DVF wraps. All the signs were there for a comeback. The question was how. The answer, it seemed at the time, was Federated Department Stores, which, after many mergers and acquisitions, had become one of the largest better retailers in America, owning Bloomingdale's and Macy's, among others. I had breakfast with Allen Questrom, the chairman, whom I had known from the old days, and I proposed designing a private label brand exclusive to his stores. It could start with dresses, and over time expand to an array of products including accessories, intimate apparel, and home furnishings. It was a bit audacious to try and sell myself to Federated considering I hadn't been in the retail world for ten years, but the idea of striking an exclusive agreement with a designer appealed to Allen.

He introduced me to his management and we discussed both the merchandising aspect and the financial side. I wanted to use the same formula as the TV shopping: I would design, and they would buy from the manufacturer and own the liability of the inventory. Since it would require a large commitment and investment on their part, I felt I should show my commitment, too. I would invest in setting up a professional design studio with experienced and talented designers. It sounded like a plan.

Without further ado, I gave up my office at Fifth Avenue and Fifty-Seventh Street, where I had been since 1979. It had shrunk from a full floor to a small corner that was outdated, inadequate, and too expensive for what it was. I needed a larger, new space that would inspire creativity—something that could be both a design studio and a showroom where we would make presentations to buyers and press.

At thirty, I had wanted a very grown-up, glamorous space uptown. Approaching fifty, I wanted something more bohemian and my own. I looked downtown and found an 1858 brick carriage house in the Meatpacking District, way, way west on Twelfth Street, very close to the Hudson River. The fifteen-thousand-square-foot space was both charming and open, with a small pool inside the entrance, exposed beams, and redbrick walls. The building had had many lives—a stable for police horses, a studio for the painter Lowell Nesbitt, and most recently the headquarters of an advertising agency.

I fell in love with it immediately, to the deep concern of Alexandre, who could not understand why I would buy a house in the smelly neighborhood of butchers, meatpackers, and prostitutes. He was so horrified that he called my mother to get her to try and talk me out of it. They failed, though there was some truth to their objections. It was smelly, and in the morning pretty bad to step around the condoms and the trash in the street. Yet I loved it. In a weird way the cobblestone streets reminded me of Belgium, and I paid no attention to the naysayers. I bought myself the carriage house for my fiftieth birthday.

In the West Village there was a lot of energy, diversity, and a sense of community I never felt on Fifty-Seventh Street. I was in a real neighborhood and quickly established relationships with my colorful neighbors. The first was Florent Morellet, the flamboyant son of the famous French painter François Morellet. Florent had a diner nearby on Gansevoort Street that was open twenty-four hours a day where local artists, workers, and drag queens ate. He often dressed in drag himself and was so upfront about being HIV positive that he posted his T-cell count next to the menu over the counter. Florent was really the godfather of the community and determined to preserve the old, low-brick surrounding buildings. Would I help his campaign to turn the neighborhood into a historic district by holding a fund-raiser? "Of course."

The fund-raiser, the first of many I had in the second little building I bought next to my studio, was like a fair, with a lot of local restaurants participating. It was a great success, and in 2003, Florent managed to get local legislation through to declare the neighborhood the Gansevoort Market Historic District. It was a huge accomplishment and saved the wonderful old brick buildings from the wreckers' ball. Florent turned a dream into reality. Alexandre began to appreciate the colorful eclecticism of the neighborhood and soon moved his office there into my space.

Everything seemed new and vital on West Twelfth Street, including my fledgling business. From the moment we moved in, everything seemed to go faster and grow larger—the pressure and stress along with it.

The team was small. Kathy and Colleen handled all of the Silk Assets business I still had with HSN. The design team for my new project with Federated was international: Christian from Holland, Evelyn from Puerto Rico, and Sergio from Colombia. Alexandra, my son's new bride, who had studied fashion at the Parsons School of Design, joined us. Her first role was to go through the prints. Just as I had done decades ago at Ferretti's factory, she came quietly into the studio and began sorting through the archived prints from my early years. Together, we created the first designs during the months we were still negotiating with Federated.

I felt the need to recreate the jersey I had used for my dresses in the seventies. Ferretti had died and his factories were closed, but I had kept swatches of the fabrics. After Ferretti and I parted ways in 1979, a certain Mr. Lam in Hong Kong produced my dresses for Carl Rosen and Puritan Fashions.

I hadn't see Mr. Lam in almost fifteen years when I visited him in Hong Kong to talk to him about re-creating my Italian jersey from the seventies. His factory had been small when I'd last seen him. Now his factories were very large and my business very small, yet he welcomed me with open arms. In return for the investment he would have to make to develop my signature fabric and set up better print-ing facilities, I moved the production of Silk Assets to his factories. He put his technical people at my disposal and together we developed the perfect jersey fabric, as tight as the original Italian one but this time 100 percent silk and more luxurious. I also shared my knowledge about hand printing, and spent long hours with their technicians. The process took a lot of patience and determination, but it was worth it for sure. The results were astounding.

Working hands-on in Mr. Lam's factories, I felt I had gone back in time, except now I was in China eating noodles with the workers for lunch and not in Italy eating spaghetti. It was exhausting going back and forth from Mr. Lam's office in Hong Kong to the factories in China, accompanied by Patso, his right hand. She worked just as hard, totally committed to what we were trying to do.

Another part of my investment was to write a business memoir to draw a line between the present and future, and introduce myself to new customers. Without hesitation, I went to my friend Linda Bird Francke, who had played such a big part in my life with her articles in *New York* magazine and *Newsweek*, to help me write the book. I would time the publication of *Diane: A Signature Life* to coincide with the launch of my first collection for Federated. The plan was to do personal appearances in their stores across the country, promoting the book and the clothes. I was close to finishing the book in the summer of 1996 when the crushing news came in: the deal with Federated had fallen through.

I got the call in my car on a Friday afternoon, while driving to the country. Allen Questrom, the chairman, had left the company. The col-laboration no longer seemed right for them. They were sorry. I'm sure there were other reasons, too, but if they ever told me, I've forgotten them. I was in total shock. I was devastated. I had counted so much on this arrangement. What was I going to do?

That weekend Barry was with me in Cloudwalk. As usual, he reassured me and encouraged me to move on. By Monday morning, I had a new plan. An obvious plan. One that had been under my nose the whole time. The wrap dress. My quintessential symbol of the seventies. I would relaunch the wrap and once again I would do it on my own.

There were many positive signs. The success of QVC had made my name extremely well known again; I was surprised to see how high I ranked in a poll of brand-name recognition published in *Women's Wear Daily* that year. So there I was, with name recognition, a demand for the dress, and the perfect fabric at my disposal.

I called Rose Marie Bravo and my mother's adage proved right once again. One door closed. Another door opened. "How exciting," Rose Marie said. "We would be proud to launch your wrap dresses at Saks."

I had retired at thirty-six, and here I was beginning again, at fifty. I was nervous but it was unbelievably exciting. Reintroducing my brand successfully in a high-end department store like Saks would prove to the world, and to myself, that the first time hadn't been an accident. But first I had to make it happen.

I decided to call the new line "Diane," the same name I had used, with a label in my handwriting, for my short-lived couture line. That label also became the first new print I designed: an allover "Diane" signature print. The idea had come to me while I was talking on the phone, looking at the label and doodling on a piece of paper. All those intertwined "Dianes" looked very much like the original prints and felt right. That led me to rework the original twig print by adding more colors. I reissued the original wood print and added a few new ones, all geometric and bold in the style of the seventies.

The announcement of my exclusive arrangement with Saks set off an enormous buzz about the return of the wrap, and me! Newspapers and magazines revisited my marriage to Egon, the children, and the phenomenon of the wrap. The *International Herald Tribune* described the dress as "The Image of an Era," over the subhead, "The Charmed Lives and Free Spirit of Diane von Furstenberg." The *New York Times Magazine* saw me as a fairy tale—"Once upon a time, there was a princess with an idea. The idea was a dress"—and *Women's Wear Daily* really got it right: "Diane's Wild Ride."

Beginning again made me feel young and fearless, but, looking back, my diary of that year also reveals many fears. As usual, I did not show my insecurities. I sounded full of confidence in all the interviews I gave, but it was a complicated time for me. On the one hand, I felt excited and rejuvenated, restarting the adventure of the wrap dress, flattered by the reaction of young girls and the excitement of Rose Marie Bravo. On the other hand, I was scared and constantly questioning myself. I did not feel secure. I was going ahead but I was afraid to fail. My rejection by Federated had left me off-balance in my business life and I was also living a major rejection in my private life: Mark Peploe had left me for another woman and I was hurting. What a strange time it was. Part of me felt old and for the first time ever, on a trip to LA, I consulted a few cosmetic surgeons. Those visits made me feel even more scared, insecure, and confused, although I did know that cosmetic surgery was not the solution. I did, however, get my teeth fixed; I'd had problems since a bad fall when I was ten years old, and seven weeks of radiation made the situation much worse.

Alexandra introduced me to her dentist, Dr. Irwin Smigel, and after months of work he left me with two gifts: a beautiful smile for the first time in my life, and the phone number for Tracie Martyn.

The launch at Saks was set for September 1997, and during the summer countdown there were a few unexpected and very welcome confidence boosters. I went to an elegant wedding of friends of my children, in Virginia, where all the young girls were wearing the "it" Tocca dresses: simple, colorful shifts by the then very popular Dutch designer Marie-Anne Oudejans. However the young hip Marie-Anne herself had asked to borrow a sample of a new DVF wrap in the beige-and-white signature print, and to my delight, she wore it to the wedding. I was extremely flattered. It meant a lot.

I got another boost in July at the Dior couture show in Paris. I'd brought a new wrap dress with me and wore it, a choice that was equally daring and nerve-racking. Here I was in the most sophisticated circumstances, a Dior couture show in an elegant greenhouse, wearing a dress that was basically the same as I would have worn twenty years before. But amazingly, it was that little dress that created a buzz in Paris and caught the attention of Amy Spindler, the talented young fashion editor at the *New York Times*.

"She slipped one on for John Galliano's Christian Dior couture show in July in Paris, over a bathing suit," Amy wrote for the Sunday *New York Times Magazine*. "By the time the sun began blazing through the roof, everyone near her was envying her wrap: She pulled the skirt aside to reveal leg, pushed up the sleeves to reveal arms, and was left with a dress the size of the bathing suit beneath. Actresses Rita Wilson and Kate Capshaw, seated across from her, raved about her look. So did the models backstage. And that was when she knew." I did know it was happening but it was still unbelievable. "Oh, I'd like a dress like that," one model after another said to me as they stood in their beautiful ball gowns when I was taken backstage to see John Galliano. There was such enthusiasm for the dress in Paris that I called my office in New York to arrange for more samples to be brought over by a friend so I could wear another wrap to the Chanel couture show. I wore a different print every day.

Amy was just as enthusiastic back in New York at the first, unconventional fashion show I gave on West Twelfth Street in September. It was only wrap dresses and a few beaded printed shirts over white pants. The models came down the carriage house's steep, narrow spiral staircase onto a carpet I'd designed for the little runway that was printed with the black-and-white "Diane" signature print. Looking back, I cannot believe that at age fifty I was once again a little do-it-yourself start-up. It was not so different from my first show at the Gotham Hotel. I was following my instinct, determined to make it work. The press loved it, including Amy.

"Yes, yes, yes, Diane Von Furstenberg's bold bias-cut wrap dress is back," she wrote in the *Times*. "Redesigned for the 90's, it is sleek and sexy, but still a dress with a sassy mom quality." I cannot calculate how much I owe to Amy. The influential fashion reporter, who wore the dresses herself, was such an editorial supporter that she became as important to the new line as Diana Vreeland had been to the original wrap. (Sadly, Amy died of cancer in 2004. She was only forty.)

I needed to find the right image, with the right spirit, for the first ad campaign for Saks. I went to my friend, French photographer Bettina Rheims, who is a master at photographing women, and we chose Danielle Zinaich to be our girl. Danielle was in her late twenties, had great legs and perfect body language. Her brown hair was shoulder length and her face quite long and distinctive, but what we loved most about her was her personality and her huge laugh that revealed her prominent gums shamelessly. Danielle and I flew to Paris and we shot the relaunch of the wrap dress in my Left Bank apartment. Most of the shoot was in vivid color, except for one dress that we photographed in black-and-white. I had no idea how fortuitous that would be.

The problem arose when I proudly called Rose Marie Bravo to my studio to see the edgy photos that Bettina and I had done in Paris. She and I were accomplices in this venture, relaunching the wrap, but she didn't like the pictures at all. She found them too hard, too decadent, too reminiscent of a recent controversy: "heroin-chic" images of pale, ill-looking models. I was devastated. All those beautiful photos in vivid colors rejected. Rose Marie must have felt sorry for me because on her way out, she pointed at the black-and-white photos of Danielle, one serious and one laughing, showing her exaggerated gums and declared, "Use these. She looks happy!"

I stared at those two black-and-white pictures for hours after Rose Marie left. I didn't know what to do after spending so much time and money with Bettina shooting hundreds of images for the beautiful color ads, but I had to do something. And then it came to me. "I'll make them speak," I said to myself, "and give them a reason to be." I put them next to each other and under the serious shot of Danielle, I wrote "He stared at me all night" and under the laughing one, I wrote "And then he said, 'Something about you reminds me of my mother.'"

The copy was funny but also risky, leading people at my office to call it ridiculous. "Nobody wants to look like their mother," they said. But I thought it was provocative and I liked it, and more to the point, so did Rose Marie, who agreed to endorse the campaign, which turned out to be very successful.

We launched at Saks in New York on September 9 with great fanfare. Television cameras and print photographers crowded around the women standing in line in the dress department, many with their daughters, to buy the new dresses. The demand was so great the dresses quickly sold out and the women who had to go home without one put their names on waiting lists for the next shipment. "It feels like déjà vu," I kept telling the hordes of press. They saw explosive success that looked familiar, but I meant it also as a cautionary tale.

Once again I was on a runaway train without a business plan or a strategy. I didn't even have a president to manage the new company. There'd been no time. Our new West Twelfth Street studio was still in disarray. I hadn't finished renovating it, there weren't enough phone lines, and the computers kept crashing. I remember feeling distracted and exhausted during the launch at Saks, a state exacerbated by my return to the fitting rooms with the customers and seeing my face twenty years older looking back at me in the mirrors. Still, the return of the wrap was a dream come true.

Alexandra and I toured the country, making personal appearances at the Saks stores from coast to coast selling the dresses with lots of hype. We got a lot of press—a beautiful new von Furstenberg princess in one wrap, her mother-in-law in another—illustrating the ageless-ness of the dress. The dresses sold well when we were in the stores, but the excitement, and sales, didn't hold after we left. The reintroduction of the wrap started like a big soufflé, and the soufflé fell flat. I didn't know what to do. "Business hard, losing money, no plan," I wrote in my journal.

I had been out of the stores for so long that I didn't know the new reality: Young girls in the nineties rarely shopped in the dress depart-ment, and that is where we were placed at Saks. The older generation still shopped there, but Alexandra and her friends bought their clothes at smaller boutiques. And that's where the wrap dress, newly and more sleekly designed, was truly reborn.

Scoop. What would we have done without Scoop? Owned by a friend of Alexandra's, Scoop was a very hip, new little shop on Broadway, way downtown in SoHo, where just about everything they sold was black, including the combat boots. But Scoop's owner, Stefani Greenfield, loved the colorful new wraps and simply hung them on hangers in her window. They sold out in half an hour. She couldn't keep them in stock with the huge demand from the downtown girls—and soon from the uptown girls when Scoop opened another shop on Third Avenue in the seventies. Where young people shopped, the dresses sold at meteoric speed, but it was just not the case in the old-fashioned dress departments we were also counting on.

At the beginning of 1998, I hired Susan Falk, the former president of Henri Bendel, to be my president. We also hired a well-known consulting company to advise us on what distribution channel we should pursue. Susan introduced me to Catherine Malandrino, a talented young French designer with whom she had worked previously. Catherine came to see me at the Carlyle, where I was living at the time. We talked about her journey as a designer and I showed her my newest wrap in a dark-green camouflage leopard print. She loved it and agreed to join us.

We introduced new wraps, and some simple solid-color dresses with soft drape, to the buyers by staging a presentation that was inspired by the old Paris couture houses. I transformed the studio into a living room, decorating it with the sofa, some paintings, a huge mirror, and a piano from my old Fifth Avenue apartment. Every fifteen minutes or so, models would appear in different designs and strike motionless poses by the piano or around the indoor pool as the pianist played Gershwin or Joplin.

Catherine brought a lot of value to the fledgling company. I wore one of her designs myself the following year when I sat for my portrait by Francesco Clemente on the day Talita was born. I remember joking about being a sexy grandmother as I posed for Francesco that day. The painting hangs now in the lobby of my studio on Fourteenth Street and will be forever in my memory as the day I become a grandmother for the first time. That dress was called Angelina and was cleverly draped and very flattering with all kinds of details from old-fashioned dressmaking. Angelina proved to be very successful.

Alexandra was getting more and more involved and was a wonderful image for the company. Though she liked the new draped dresses well enough, she was still concerned about our lack of direction. She had a point. Between the wraps and the new drape dresses we clearly had a viable collection but we didn't have a clear path of how to distribute it and move the business forward. The consultants we had hired advised us to go into the moderate market, but it didn't match the sophistication of the designs. I was confused and stressed.

That summer as I was driving to Teterboro Airport in New Jersey to meet Barry and fly to Alaska, I took a very bad turn. Having passed the airport turnoff, I swerved, bumped into something, and was spun back onto the highway where I hit an eighteen-wheeler. I had a big, huge pain in my chest and I remember asking the ambulance crew, "Can you live if you have a hole in your heart?" It turned out that in addition to the eighteen stitches I needed in my head, I had broken five or six ribs and punctured a lung. (I also totaled Barry's BMW.)

I spent the next two painful but peaceful weeks in a small hospital in Hackensack, New Jersey, with great doctors and such tight security that I was convinced there was a mob boss on my floor. Barry and the children wanted desperately for me to be transferred to a hospital in New York, but I refused. I loved that little hospital and I loved the time alone, as Hackensack was far enough from Manhattan to discourage visitors. I needed a break. I knew I was exhausted and confused, and so did Alexandre. "You had the accident because you don't know what you're doing," he said, not as a reproach but out of concern. That was perhaps a harsh comment, but I think he was totally right. Just as a few years before I'd thought my tongue cancer symbolized my inability to express myself, I saw the accident as a symptom of my lack of a road map for my business.

The nights were long and painful in the hospital, despite my wonderful nurse with whom I became friends. I have few memories of those two weeks in a no-man's-land, as I never wrote about it in my diaries. All I know is that I had a tube in my lung, did not read or watch television, and waited motionless for my body to heal. It did. Slowly and steadily I sweated out all the bad.

I knew I had to make a change and the catalyst presented itself the moment I arrived back at my apartment in the Carlyle—and discovered water pouring into the bedroom from a leak in the ceiling. "That's it," I said to myself. "I'm moving downtown."

And another new life began.

I created a wonderful living space next to my private office on the top floor of the West Twelfth Street studio carriage house. I decorated the living area with Balinese artifacts and put an iron canopy bed against the exposed brick wall. I made a large dressing room that was also a yoga studio. I loved the décor of my new bohemian lifestyle, so different from the Carlyle. In the morning I would make a cup of coffee and cross the highway practically in my pajamas to walk along the river. I had a small guest room where my mother stayed when she visited me. She was never really comfortable there; years later it occurred to me that the exposed brick may have reminded her of the camps.

On the other hand, Christian Louboutin loved staying in that guest room and practically lived there as he showed his early collections of shoes on my dining room table. At the time he had just begun selling his sexy, red-soled heels to Barneys, Jeffrey, and Neiman Marcus. As I watched him develop new, spectacular shoes every season, selling only a few styles at a time, I suggested he build a core line he could offer every season, and was proud that I was able to help him build his talent into a huge global brand. We became the best of friends, going on to share personal appearances across the country, and began taking lots of holidays together. We've walked and driven the dusty Silk Road in Uzbekistan all the way from Tashkent to Samarkand, Bukhara, Khiva, and Fergana, to end up on the border of Afghanistan. Christian and I are both Capricorns, and like two little goats we love to climb. We've hiked up and down the hills of Egypt and the steep mountains of Bhutan.

What I loved most of all about my West Twelfth Street carriage house was the feeling that I belonged there. My personal style and designs were one and the same again—simple, happy, sexy—and everything in my life was beginning to feel coherent for the first time in years. All of this, including the creative characters in my vibrant neighborhood, made me feel like a young new me. Once again I was giving lots of fun parties, including one for the publication of *Signature Life*. Tatiana asked a friend of a friend to organize the music, and that is when we all met Russell Steinberg, who soon after became father of my second grandchild, Antonia.

The business was still limping along, but little by little we were gaining traction and I was certainly happier than I'd been in a while.

I was very touched and proud when the CFDA asked me to join its board of directors in 1999. It was very reassuring to be recognized by my colleagues. For the first time in many years, I no longer felt like an outsider. I was back in the world of fashion.

What I didn't anticipate was a run-in I had with Alexandre in what has become known as the "family intervention." The whole family was gathered in Barry's office in New York where we were discussing the creation of the Diller–von Furstenberg Family Foundation for charitable donations. After that discussion, Alexandre, who manages our family money, confronted me. "You've got to refocus your energies on making a plan for what you want to do with the company and stop hemorrhaging money," he said. "Or else pull the plug."

I was very angry at being confronted like that—or being confronted at all, for that matter. It was my money after all, and there was progress. I did understand Alex's concern, but in my mind, this time it was less about money and more about me. When I'd first started out in business, my goal had been financial independence and I had achieved it. This time my goal was to prove to myself and the world that the first time around hadn't been a fluke. My pride was more important than the cost of achieving that goal. It was also about the wrap dress, the style that was mine and had a place in women's closets again. Pull the plug? Now?

I slammed my fist down hard on the table. "Give me six months!" I said. "I'll turn it around. You'll see." Alex backed off and we all agreed to the six months.

He was right, of course. I couldn't just keep spending money without a plan. But I felt I might be on my way with the enthusiasm of young women for my dresses again, and that's what I wanted to work on. I did, however, need professional sales help.

And that's when Paula Sutter came into my life.

Stefani from Scoop introduced me to Paula, her young friend and former colleague, over lunch at Balthazar, the French downtown bistro. Paula, who was then greatly pregnant, had been the vice president of sales and marketing for DKNY. She and Stefani had both been part of Donna Karan's dream team that was so successful in the eighties launching DKNY. Many of the women on that team went on to have spectacular careers. "You should hire her," Stefani said. It was I who had to do the convincing when Paula visited me in my office. She didn't want to commit to a full-time job because of her impending motherhood, but I managed to persuade her to come on as a part-time consultant. That was 1998. When Susan Falk, who wanted to return to corporate life, left the following year, Paula became president of Diane von Furstenberg Studio. She remained the company's invaluable president for fourteen years.

It was a struggle for her at first, accentuated when Alexandre came to see Paula to reissue his now familiar ultimatum. "You've got six months to turn a profit or close it down," he told her. Not a great welcome. Paula, however, was on my side.

With her credentials she could have gone to bigger, more successful names at the time, but she saw that our company had really good DNA and really good bones but needed "Windexing," as she put it, to get rid of the messiness. She was as excited as I was about the possibilities that lay in the young, not in the middle-aged dress department. The demographic model had been wrong from the start, so we changed course.

The retail experience was trending toward a new, more modern approach. Department stores were beginning to establish contemporary or "affordable luxury" divisions and that's where Paula thought we belonged. It would be a great opportunity for us to go after the younger consumer and pretty much retell our story in a new and modern way, but to get there, we first we had to reposition the brand as universally cool.

Paula was enthusiastic and determined. She had such energy talking to the luxury stores like Bergdorf Goodman, but it was difficult. My name was "polluted" they claimed because we were still selling on television, and some buyers still thought of me as an old brand even though by that time we had an enviable track record with contemporary girls. The signature label, Diane, was also problematic. They thought it old-fashioned. Luckily an old boyfriend, Craig Brown, the graphic designer who made the Rolling Stone logo of Mick Jagger's tongue, reappeared in my life at that moment and he redesigned the label as a typeface "Diane von Furstenberg."

We took other steps as well. "Diane von Furstenberg Silk Assets" became "Silk Assets." I eased myself out of the HSN broadcasts and Alicia, a young woman from the office, replaced me.

Paula established monthly deliveries to create an ongoing fresh flow of merchandise in the stores. For our next press day I had the idea of creating evocative *tableaux vivants* around the studio's pool illustrating the themes of those monthly deliveries: the plants, the flowers, the sea. The models were ravishing in the small, focused collection of featherweight chiffon and jersey dresses in trademark prints and matching colors. The buyers and press walked into a living painting. It was colorful, sexy, edgy, and different from what anyone else was doing at the time.

We continued our show-and-tell in Paris. We packed up and took a booth at Tranoï, an international fashion trade fair for young designers at the Carrousel du Louvre during French Market Week. The best specialty stores from around the world go there. These shops set the taste for everyone else. We were hoping to be a presence in those stores and it happened when Colette, one of the coolest shops, ordered our sexy, printed dresses for its store in Paris. It was at that time that Betsee Isenberg, the hot showroom rep in LA, also took the line on to sell on the West Coast.

Alexandre was still skeptical. We weren't really making any money, but there was definitely traction. Paula did some projections and a small business plan when we came back to New York. She showed them to Barry and Alexandre. "I understand," Barry laughed when she finished her presentation. "You want to try and give the business a blood transfusion." We adopted those words because that was exactly what we were trying to do—and six months later, it was back to Paris with the next collection.

I remember those days with tremendous affection. Five or six of us from the New York studio would pile into my apartment on the rue de Seine along with all the clothes, essentially camping there for the duration of the fair. We were a skeletal crew—Paula, of course, and Astrid, the best salesperson ever, speaking every language and trying every dress on herself. There was Maureen from marketing and Luisella, the smart Italian girl who at the time was my assistant. We laughed a lot and were very successful at getting orders in the very best international shops.

I felt young again, propelled by the girls around me, and I shared their excitement and enthusiasm. I felt their age. There were no big business meetings, no big marketing plans. None of that. The second time started just as organically as the first. It was, after all, a small business. It was really like incubating a new, young brand and we did it on a shoestring, living off my profit from HSN.

Soon we were selling, selling, selling to specialty stores in England, France, Italy, Spain—all over Europe—as well as shops in the US. Scoop was, of course, our mainstay in New York, and in LA it was Fred Segal, the brilliant retailer who had been the first, in the sixties, to open a denim-only store. Both stores were big fans of the brand and getting the word out through their very loyal client base. Relaunching amid the nostalgia for the seventies turned out to be perfect. Colette loved paying glamour homage to the seventies and Studio 54, all of which I had thoroughly lived. That I was an original player of the time gave authenticity to my clothes, interviews, and personal appearances. There we were in our booth at the fair, right beside the cool, young designers, and it was all encouraging, but the income was still small.

I looked for a shortcut. On a flight from London to New York I sat next to Tom Ford, and he expressed great interest in what I was doing. I had a flash: Why not sell a piece of the company to Gucci to raise some money so we could go on smoothly? A few months later I flew to London with Barry and Alexandre and Paula met us there. It was the summer of 1999 and Barry was involved in a huge deal trying to buy up Universal, but he took the time to come with us to Gucci. Our meeting didn't get off to a great start. Tom and his partner Domenico De Sole were late, and Barry was upset. Nonetheless, we went ahead with our presentation and they seemed interested. We had several meetings with their people in New York over the next few months, but somehow shortcuts don't work for me. In the end, they were not interested and invested in Stella McCartney instead. I was disappointed.

In the midst of all this, Catherine Malandrino left us to develop her own line and open her own shop. In came Nathan Jenden in 2001. He stayed with me for almost ten years.

Nathan was English, thirty I think at the time, and had worked with John Galliano and Tommy Hilfiger so he understood both high fashion and Main Street, and he had a little funky side. I liked him from the beginning when I'd asked him to make a presentation (which he promptly lost but found again) and he came back with a sketch of a girl wearing a crossword puzzle print dress that he titled The Rebel Princess. When he came into my office he was impressed by the numbers of books I had around me, and I was impressed that he'd noticed them.

Nathan brought a lot of feng shui and a little rock 'n' roll to the clothes and we had a great run together. Nathan was incredibly talented and he was able to create magic during fittings with his aggressive scissors. The first show we did together happened two days before 9/11, which left us all in a state of shock and disarray. His work was so sharp, it managed to keep our numbers up as the city's economy took a huge hit. That year he came we also opened our first shop in New York next door to the carriage house. It was a tiny boutique you could barely find. Calvin Klein came to the opening of my hidden-away shop and looked at the little dresses. "What a wonderful concept," he said. Coming from Calvin, who doesn't like color or print, that was a huge compliment. I was really beginning to feel on a high, even though Gucci had rejected me.

The high continued in Los Angeles at the Academy Awards. Barry and I have always given a Saturday picnic lunch for our friend Graydon Carter, the editor of *Vanity Fair* and host of its longtime Oscar party. A lot of beautiful stars come to our lunch and more and more started arriving in DVF. Now we were definitely gaining ground!

From just a few little dresses, we expanded into a full collection. Twice a year we held formal runway shows at our studio. The names—Working Girl, Under the Volcano, Rebel Princess—reflected the easy, sexy, independent, on-the-go, slightly mischievous woman we designed for. After the successful Dolce Diva fashion show, a light fell and hurt two editors. I felt terribly guilty. I visited Hilary Alexander, the highly respected editor of the *Daily Telegraph* in the hospital and she was an incredible sport. In spite of her injury, she gave us a great review, but the time had come to join the big leagues and show in the official New York Fashion Week tents.

By 2002 we were in virtually every quality department store, including the grande dame of them all, Bergdorf Goodman. I let my hair go curly again. The Comeback Kid had arrived! In three amazing years, I had gone from losing money, and being advised by my concerned family to shut down, to being very profitable. No one in the industry could believe it. No one expected us to do what we did, and a lot of people were surprised by how we were able to reinvent the brand. Paula and I positioned the business in a very modern way, and here we were—a 1970s business that had successfully transitioned into the twenty-first century with the original centerpiece dress surrounded by new, multigenerational global designs.

We grew as opportunities arose, without a master plan. We opened a shop in Miami in 2003, and the next year in London in a little boutique in Notting Hill, where we were hot, hot, hot. Paris followed the next year, with a spectacular launch. Madonna happened to be in Paris so I sent her an email. She came to the opening with her daughter and a retinue of paparazzi and bought a wrap that she wore at a press conference she gave in Israel. You can't ask for a better friend or better publicity than that!

Madonna came through again a few years later in Los Angeles at the 2008 Oscar after-party she cohosted with Demi Moore. They surprised me by wearing the same gold wrap dress the stylist Rachel Zoe had ordered for them from my spring fashion show! I really felt that as a designer, I had arrived. I was exhilarated that same night by the commercial American Express ran twice during the Oscars broadcast. They had commissioned Bennett Miller, the Academy Award–nominated director, to do it, and we shot at Cloudwalk and at the studio. Bennett refused to have me read a script; he interviewed me instead, and used that for the voice-over. That night millions of people heard me say: *I didn't really know what I wanted to do, but I knew the woman I wanted to become.* Even though I must have said that sentence many times before, hearing it on TV made me realize its power. That desire is the spirit of my brand.

Over the next few years we opened shops in Tokyo, Jakarta, St. Tropez, Brussels, Shanghai, Hong Kong, Moscow, Madrid, second and third shops in Paris, São Paulo, Beijing. Opening the shop in Antwerp, run by my sister-in-law, was particularly rewarding because it was my first store in Belgium. Axel Vervoordt, the renowned architect and interior designer, gave a big, beautiful dinner for me in his castle; for the first time ever, I felt recognized as a designer in my native country.

Moscow presented another wonderful opportunity. Our collection in 2005 was Russian-inspired and was carried by a shop called Garderobe that invited me to Moscow. They held a little fashion show and dinner for me at Tolstoy's house on the Ulitsa Lva Tolstogo! After the show, sitting in Tolstoy's garden under the lilac trees, drinking champagne and giving interviews made me think how thrilled my Russian father would have been.

Another great memory is the visit to Cloudwalk by Roberto Stern, the Brazilian jewelry designer who co-owns and runs the jewelry company H. Stern. I had always wanted to design fine jewelry and had approached his father, Hans, thirty years earlier to collaborate. I loved the quality of their jewelry, but Hans had turned me down.

I had tried again with the son in 2001, but again not much happened. Roberto, I found out later, had been a little bit intimidated by me at our first meetings, but intimidation turned to inspiration during his visit to Cloudwalk, and we entered into a wonderful collaboration. He did a phenomenal job of interpreting my vision and was not afraid to make the really bold jewelry I love—huge, crystal rings and the heavy, 18-karat yellow-gold Sutra link bracelet that I wear every day, each link engraved with one of my favorite sutras: Harmony, Integrity, Peace, Abundance, Love, Knowledge, Laughter, and Creativity.

The business was growing so rapidly the carriage house on West Twelfth Street filled, then overflowed with staff. The DVF family had outgrown our home and we needed more room.

I bought two historic buildings on the corner of Washington and Fourteenth Street, still in the Meatpacking District. Part of the buildings had been used by John Jacob Astor as housing for his workers. It took three years to build a new six-story headquarters and studio because we were in a historic district, which I'd helped create via the first benefit I'd held on West Twelfth Street six years before. Instead of tearing the buildings down to create my new headquarters, I had to go to the landmarks commission and present a wildly expensive plan to preserve the two brick façades, gut the interior, and build from within. I even created a bedroom, however eccentric it might seem to sleep in a glass tree house on the roof. West Twelfth Street turned out to have been a wise investment, despite all the resistance I'd faced. I'd bought the two carriage houses for $5 million in 1997. I sold them in 2003 for $20 million.

All this growth was boosting my confidence, which is vital to how you view opportunities. My self-assurance was reinforced in 2005 when I received the CFDA's Lifetime Achievement Award, then again when the next year I was elected president of the CFDA. Recognition by peers is the most valid recognition, and without it I doubt I would have undertaken the most audacious challenge of all, China.

"I want to be "known in China." These words topped my New Year's Resolutions on the eve of 2010, and I take resolutions seriously since New Year's Eve is also my birthday. It was a huge goal, of course, but it was a goal to make happen.

I have always been fascinated with China. I had been there many times, starting in 1989 when there were barely any cars in the streets. I had made friends in Beijing and Shanghai over the years: artists, writers, businesspeople. Suddenly everybody was looking at China as a great business opportunity, but I didn't want to be just another opportunistic brand. I wanted to understand their culture as well as explain my own. By being the face of my brand from the beginning, I'd always had a relationship with my customers, an understanding, and I wanted to do the same in China.

I had a way: the exhibit of my work, life, and art that I'd already mounted in Moscow and São Paulo to introduce myself to the markets there. Bill Katz, who designs exhibitions and interiors and is a longtime friend, suggested an extraordinary venue: Pace Beijing, the largest privately owned art gallery in the world. Arne Glimcher, the gallery's owner, enthusiastically agreed to host the show.

I was so excited. Others were not. Paula was against my China campaign; by this time Nathan had left and Yvan Mispelaere had joined as creative director. There was a lot to do, and he needed to be fully briefed and integrated into the company. Furthermore, she argued—legitimately—that it was premature to do an exhibition in China. Our presence in mainland China was limited to two stores in Beijing and one in Shanghai, and from a business perspective, mounting the exhibit wouldn't justify the huge commitment of money, time, and effort from the company. "Wait a few years until we're better established in China," Paula said. But my instinct told me the timing was right and I insisted on pressing ahead. The opening for the six-week exhibition was set for April 4, 2011.

I explained the Beijing exhibition to friends at a dinner given for me in Shanghai by Pearl Lam, the flamboyant art dealer. "What about Shanghai?" they asked. They were eager for me to do something in their city. "Give a ball," suggested Wendi Deng Murdoch, then the wife of media mogul Rupert Murdoch. "No one in China gives a ball." My Chinese friends loved the idea and so did I. "We'll call it the Red Ball," I decided.

The next day I visited the celebrated artist Zhang Huan in his cavernous pipe-factory-turned-studio in an industrial suburb of Shanghai. From the first moment, I knew it would be the perfect venue for a ball—much more interesting than any grand hotel. Zhang loved the idea, which in turn delighted the Shanghainese, who have an informal rivalry with their counterparts in Beijing. The Red Ball would be March 31, four days before the opening of the retrospective.

We expected seven hundred guests at the ball but more than a thousand came. It was a who's who of Chinese talent, including the Academy Award–winning composer Tan Dun (*Crouching Tiger, Hidden Dragon*), the multi-award-winning actress Zhang Ziyi (*Crouching Tiger, 2046*), China's beautiful top international model Du Juan, and many, many others. I wore a sequined gown with the Chinese character for love on the bodice, and I really did love that spectacular evening. So did the hordes of Chinese press. My Chinese partners, David and Linda Ting and Michael and Jess Wang, were ecstatic.

People in China are still talking about the DVF Red Ball, I am told by my friend Hung Huang, the highly influential author, blogger, the founder of the magazine *iLook* and the first Chinese designer store, BNC. Scores of masked men dressed in black manipulating red laser beams around the thirty-foot-high studio, Zhang Huan's Ming dynasty temple floating on red mist, Jin Xing's modern dance troupe snapping giant red fans in the temple and performing to kettle drums, the after-dinner disco amid spinning lights and a red glitter floor—all brilliantly designed by my friend Alex de Betak, the magician who designs the sets of my fashion shows.

I was so proud that night, especially because my entire family was with me: children and grandchildren, cousins, and Philippe who came from Belgium with his family. "What do you like best about your job, Didi?" Tatiana's daughter, Antonia, had asked me the day before the Red Ball. "What I like best about my job is the fact that I can dream of something and make it happen," I replied. That trip was even more special because Tatiana shot the DVF ad campaign and a spectacular film, both titled "Rendezvous," at Zhang Huan's studio in Shanghai.

Four days after the ball, a thousand people came to the opening at Pace Beijing. Chinese people were fascinated by my journey in New York in the seventies and the Andy Warhol portraits, such a contrast to where China was in the 1970s. I also commissioned four new portraits by leading Chinese artists, Arne Glimcher's idea.

Each time I walk into my office and see the ash painting Zhang Huan did of me, or into my library at Cloudwalk, where there's a portrait by Li Songsong, I'm glad I followed my instinct; they are masterpieces. I also achieved my New Year's Resolution. We have twenty-one stores in China and plans to open fourteen more in the next four years. And I am certainly "known." When I started working on the China project, I had no followers on Sina Weibo, China's version of Twitter. After the Red Ball and the exhibition, the numbers grew to three hundred thousand. As I write this, my followers have grown to over two million!

We were all on a high when we left China. We had succeeded beyond our wildest dreams, and the DVF team had performed magnificently. Little did I know that within three years, we'd be mounting

the exhibition yet again, this time in Los Angeles. It would be different though. I'd pushed alone against my team's resistance to make the
China campaign happen. When we returned to New York, I realized
making those solo decisions was a bad habit. So many things had to
change. It was time for the business to enter a third phase, a phase I
would call The New Era. The change was not easy for any of us.

6

THE NEW ERA

The realization had begun before the trip to China. Change, both exciting and painful, was in the air. Paula and I had been like Thelma and Louise, hurtling cross-country beautifully for ten years. We were the pretty girls on the block. The brand was young again, a shining star in fifty-five countries. We had opened fifty of our own shops. We had brought the business from nothing to $200 million in sales. Now what?

My goals had shifted. No longer was I striving to be financially independent. I was. I didn't need to prove that the first time around wasn't an accident. I had. What I wanted now was to turn a good company into a great company, to leave a legacy, something that would live beyond me. I had reached the age where you begin to think about what you leave your grandchildren and their children.

I was already building a legacy outside the business. Having empowered myself, it was my duty to empower other women. That is why I got involved with Vital Voices and established the DVF Awards. It was also my turn to support the fashion and New York communities that had given me so much. In fashion, the opportunity came from the CFDA. I can't overstate how honored I was to be elected its president in 2006. *Women's Wear Daily* put my election on the front cover: "Von Furstenberg Elected: Brings Power Contacts, Jet-Set Savvy to CFDA." Steven Kolb, the new executive director, and I became a team. My first goal was to turn the organization into a family, bring in fresh blood, and make sure the more established designers helped and mentored the newer ones. Together we would have more power, more leverage than on our own. The first month I was elected, Steven and I flew to Washington, DC, to lobby Congress for copyright protection against design piracy. When we arrived that morning, our lobbyist, Liz Robbins, told us it was a bad day. Everyone was busy and we would probably spend hours waiting and meet no one. To her surprise and our delight, it turned out we had more clout than she had thought. We met with Senators Hillary Clinton, John McCain, Olympia Snow, Charles Schumer, Dianne Feinstein, and Representative Nancy Pelosi, the future Speaker. We explained the urgent need to protect our designs, posed for photos, and left excited. We have yet to pass the law, but we certainly raised the profile of design and showed mass merchants the value of hiring designers instead of simply copying them.

After the disaster of 9/11 and its effect on the New York economy, my friend Anna Wintour, the powerful editor of *Vogue*, had the idea of creating a fund to identify and promote young American designers. The CFDA/Vogue Fashion Fund was created and being part of it is one of my biggest sources of pride. Some of today's brightest talents and most successful businesses have emerged from the fund. Alexander Wang, Proenza Schouler, Rodarte, Rag and Bone, Prabal Gurung, Joseph Altuzarra, Jennifer Meyer—to name just a few—all came up through it.

CFDA is committed to promoting diversity and protecting the health and well-being of models. It supports Made in NY, an initiative spearheaded by Andrew Rosen (son of Carl who saved my business in 1979) to reenergize the local garment industry. CFDA helps develop American design talent with many scholarship programs. It also rallies in times of need. We raised over one million dollars for Haiti's earthquake relief and support the Born Free campaign to eliminate the transmission of HIV from mothers to babies.

Steven and I will never forget the day we went to City Hall to meet with the newly elected mayor Michael Bloomberg. "What can the city do for fashion?" he asked. "We need a place for our fashion shows, we need a fashion center. I would love to get one of the piers along the Hudson River," I told him presumptuously.

We never got a pier, but the mayor's deputy, Dan Doctoroff, did not forget my request. We will get a home for Fashion Week at Culture Shed, a new two-hundred-thousand-square-foot, highly flexible cultural institution, which will be a crossroads for the full range of creative industries. I joined the board of Culture Shed, which will stand at the northern end of the High Line, the immensely popular park that is the pride and joy of my family.

The High Line was the dream of Josh David and Robert Hammond, young neighbors from Chelsea and the West Village, who had the audacious idea of reversing one of Mayor Giuliani's last acts, signed a few days before he left office: a demolition order for the old elevated railroad that runs from Gansevoort Street to Thirty-Fourth Street. They wanted to recycle it into a park. My family joined in their dream and we succeeded, with the help of so many. The old railway was transformed by the amazing design work of James Corner Field Operations, Diller Scofido + Renfro, and Piet Oudolf, and opened in 2009. Millions of visitors and New Yorkers enjoy strolling along the beautiful, long green ribbon of wild flowers, shrubs, and grasses above the urban streets. I am one of them.

For all of this, Forbes named me one of the twenty most powerful businesswomen in the world! Yet my own business was moving along an uncharted path from one opportunity to another without a clear set of goals or much discipline. While we had been lulled by our remarkable growth, companies that had started only a few years before, but had a clear road map and were driven by smart marketing, were suddenly worth much more.

Our new creative director Yvan Mispelaere had just started, coming in with big credentials from Gucci, where he was head designer for women's wear. Gucci's designs and ours are very much in the same sexy seventies style so it seemed a perfect fit. He came to New York in 2010 to meet Paula and me and we hired him on the spot.

It started well, with a first "inspiration" walk through the streets of Paris. I took him to see an exhibition on Isadora Duncan at the Musée Bourdelle in the 15th Arrondissement, and decided to base our next spring collection on that. We called it "Goddess." It was modern but timeless, and very sexy. The prints were bold, the colors luminous, and I loved it. Our collaboration was well received and it seemed like a match made in heaven. After that first collection that we did together, I relinquished all of my design authority. I had China to take care of, and many projects that needed my time and energy.

As I spent more time working outside the studio, Yvan was left to run the design department. A perfectionist, he took his role very seriously. Everyone was intimidated by this European designer who came from Gucci and was changing everything. Yvan's idea was to divide the collection into a vintage group called "DVF 1974," add accessories to it, and create another, elevated, more designed line to exist by its side.

It sounded great in principle, but the problem was that every one of his many ideas was produced, resulting in too many products and eventually a lack of focus. I started to sense this when I went to Honolulu just before Thanksgiving in 2011 for the grand opening of my first store in Hawaii. The manager, Marilee, and my old friend Princess Dialta di Montereale had organized a fantastic party with the who's who of Honolulu. It was a glamorous evening, we sold a lot of clothes, and everyone was happy. But I felt something was wrong ... the assortment of products was overwhelming, and though it looked good and was colorful, I wondered whether that kind of output could be sustained long term.

Furthermore, when I returned to New York, I found a lot of confusion. Design had taken over so completely in less than a year that it was affecting merchandising and production. Calendars and deadlines had started to lag, making everyone nervous. I was fond of Yvan, respected his talent, and knew how hard he worked. So I would come in and out, not digging into the problems but spending my time pacifying everyone and ceding more and more authority to him. More importantly, I also ignored Paula when she said the clothes were going off brand, confusing our buyers, and our customers.

Though I hadn't yet realized the full importance of DNA and staying on brand, we started taking an inventory of the brand's assets, and our first project was to reexamine the DVF monogram. Over the years, those three letters had become so familiar that even my family calls me DVF now! Our new, brilliant graphic designer, Diego Marini, played with the *V* and the *F*, opening it up and creating a flow the monogram had never had. He placed it between a scattering of lips on our shopping bag and stationery. I loved this bold, elegant new image that represents all I endorse: strength, love, and freedom.

I remember taking an early-morning helicopter from Cloudwalk to a windy runway at a deserted airport on Long Island in the summer of 2012. As we approached, I looked down to see our new monogram, gleaming, fifteen feet tall, surrounded by the huge team of Trey Laird, the advertising guru I had hired to shoot our next ad campaign. Designed to look metallic, and as tall as a house with nothing but sky above it and space beyond it, the logo was made almost surreal by the water we kept hosing across the ground. I loved that huge logo, and the images of our model for the season, Arizona Muse, posing in and around it. After the shoot I collapsed laughing into the juncture of the *V* and someone took a snapshot. I love that photo and fought to put it on the cover of this book!

It was a fun day. What wasn't fun was the disciplined process of creating a "brand book," a task Paula and Trey were insisting on. The goal of a brand book is to clarify what a brand stands for, to define one vision everyone can follow. At first I found this project an annoying and unnecessary exercise. But I soon realized how wrong I was when I had to struggle with the questions being posed. What is the brand? What does it stand for? What message does the brand project? Is the message consistent? What is the core design? What are the core colors? Who is the customer? Describe her. The answer to the last question should boil down to a few words, Trey said. A few words? How could forty years in fashion and millions of customers be encapsulated in a few words? Marketing genius Lapo Elkann, Alain's son, refers to my brand as the ultimate Love Brand. How could we explain that? The whole company was going through therapy and I was very stressed.

Trey was excited though. "The brand is you, it is your story. The European princess who comes to America with a few jersey dresses and turns them into an American Dream. Who else can claim that story? And your huge archive of prints, that also needs to be part of the brand book, it is unique." I decided to let him work it out.

The problems ran deeper than just improving branding and marketing. I wasn't a great manager and never will be. This became clear when Alexandre started to do a detailed audit and overview of the company. I was shocked to learn that he had trouble tracking the numbers. He was shocked by the casual and inefficient structure of the company, which was run as one entity without each division, wholesale and retail, having accountability and transparency. We'd grown fast and profitably yet we hadn't invested in the infrastructure. We didn't even have a proper CFO.

Alexandre's list of grievances was very long, yet he held some back because he didn't want to upset me. He kept on talking about transparency and accountability. I resented hearing those words but I knew he was right.

In all of my years in business I had never stuck to a business plan. I always followed my impulses and grew them into businesses. Some were huge successes, some were poorly executed and failed. That kind of energy gives authenticity and a human factor to a company, but it creates a lot of chaos, and chaos it was! Paula and I knew that if we were going to move into the big leagues, we would have to completely rework the structure, invest in experienced division heads and give them authority, add financing, and expand our family board with at least one member with a strong business and retail background.

Once I realized we desperately needed help on all levels of

management, I was shameless in seeking it. I had lunch with the chairman of Coach, the chairman of Calvin Klein, and Mickey Drexler, the retail superstar at J.Crew, among other professionals. They all said the same thing: Your name and your brand are so much bigger than your business. The growth potential is enormous. It was both frustrating and instructive—frustrating because they thought I was much bigger than I was, instructive because even though I had achieved a remarkable level of success and recognition, I was still acting like someone who was just starting.

"Build accessories," they told me. "It is critical to your growth and profitability." As it was, accessories were 10 percent of our sales, and ready-to-wear 90 percent, which had made our success to date even more astonishing. Still, to move into the next world we would have to close that gap.

Meeting these retail experts for lunch wasn't enough. I needed one on my team and on my board. We already had one board member from outside the family, Hamilton South, former president and CMO of Polo Ralph Lauren who now runs his own marketing and communications firm, HL Group. Besides being a loyal friend for over twenty years, Hamilton has an excellent strategic mind. I needed to find that trusted expertise in business as well.

During my hunt, I realized I knew the king of them all, Silas Chou. Silas is the wealthy superstar apparel investor based in Hong Kong who had bought Tommy Hilfiger some years before when the company was in trouble, then helped build it up successfully before taking it public. More recently, Silas had bought Michael Kors and done another IPO in 2011 for billions of dollars.

I knew Silas socially, and as I set out for my events in China, he had offered to give me a party at his home in Beijing to introduce me to everyone. It was a memorable dinner at his penthouse replica of a courtyard house, with a dramatic view of the Bird's Nest stadium and all across Beijing. He'd filled the apartment with celebrities and brought in dancers for the occasion. Silas also came to the Red Ball in Shanghai. He came to the exhibition in Beijing, and, back in New York, he came to lunch at my studio.

I was in awe of Silas's success in business, but he was too busy to join my board. Still, he was very enthusiastic. "You don't understand how valuable DVF is," he told me. "In order for you really to grow, Diane, you need a machine behind you. You could be so big."

"I have an idea," Tommy Hilfiger told me at yet another lunch. "Joel Horowitz. He was my partner and I owe him everything. You should meet him."

What I didn't know about Joel when he walked into my office a few weeks later in February 2012 was that he'd turned down one business idea after another that Tommy had proposed to him. He had worked hard with great success all his life, retired, and now he loved playing golf and living a pressure-free life in the Florida sun.

What I did know was that I liked him immediately, so immediately that the first thing I did was to hug him. I'd never met the man but there was something about the openness of his smile and his blue eyes.

Like the other industry professionals, he was shocked when I told him our numbers. He found them "unimaginably low" for a "lifestyle" designer, as he called me, with such recognition. "It should be a $2 billion business," he said.

Soon afterward I emailed him to ask if he could be on my board. "Yes," he replied, "I could." I immediately sent him the date of the next board meeting, and was taken aback when I got his reply: "I said I could, I didn't say I would." His loss, I thought and wrote him off.

It was Silas who got the relationship back on track when he invited Barry and me to dinner at his home in New York. Barry and I were leaving for India that night and I told Silas we couldn't stay for dinner but we'd drop in on our way to the plane. Silas took us into a side room. "I know you met with Joel Horowitz," he said. "He's your guy. You should have him on your board and make him a partner." "Really?" I said. Silas nodded. "Really," he said. "I'm going to see him next weekend and tell him." And that's how wonderful Joel joined the board and the company.

My son started to negotiate the contract with Joel over the phone in July of 2012 when we were at Herb Allen's annual conference in Sun Valley, Idaho. He didn't know I was sitting on the floor outside his door listening, my heart swelling with pride and gratitude that I had such a loving, smart son to represent the company and protect me. It turned out that Joel's hesitation was my invitation to be only a board member. "I don't do boards," he explained. "I'm not interested in giving general advice four times a year. I'd need to be an active partner." In the end, we agreed that Joel would invest for a small share of the company, my family would increase our investment, and Joel and I would cochair the board.

I was thrilled, and so was Alexandre, though for different reasons. I was excited about Joel's business expertise and Alexandre was excited that he would be an authority figure with the stature and respect to hold me in check. DVF was still reeling from the very expensive blunder I'd made the year before when I launched a new fragrance called Diane with a company too small and too inexperienced to market and distribute it properly. It was costing us a lot of money to terminate the contract. I'm sure I wouldn't have been allowed to sign with that company had Joel been there.

What was there when Joel arrived at DVF in August of 2012 was mayhem. Even thinking about it now is painful, and I blame myself. Myself only. Everyone was running around feeling my panic and the lack of direction. All along I had been trying to find solutions but there was never any time to stop and think; the bullet train just kept going.

It was during those terrible days just before the Spring 2013 collection that I finally had to confront another major problem: Our product had lost its identity. On one side the design department was making complicated fashion, while on the other side, to counterbalance it, merchandising was making banal commercial pieces. Everyone was working hard and doing what they thought was right, but truly none of it was on brand, and I didn't like any of it. My own history and the brand's heritage, the iconic dress, the archive of fifteen thousand prints—why weren't we focusing on those assets? What we had lost along the way was everything we had put in the "DVF 1974" capsule collection, which we then abandoned to address overproduction. I realized much, much later that that little capsule collection was truly the essence of the brand.

I remember those days as the worst time ever. I was going back and forth from my office to the design staging area as we prepared the fashion show, and getting more upset by the minute. Looking at racks and racks full of clothes that I knew were useless was wrenching. I couldn't sleep. I even cried. I couldn't quietly doubt anymore. It was so clear that the product was wrong. Only the beautiful colors—Yvan is a genius with colors—felt on brand but that was not enough. Still the show had to go on.

The unexpected gift that turned out to save that show was the debut of the wearable computer: Google Glass. Two months before, at the Sun Valley conference, the cofounder of Google, Sergey Brin, had called to me from where he was hiding behind a tree. He didn't want to be seen as he was wearing his new, very secret technology: glasses that were capable of taking pictures and videos and displaying email. There was a minicomputer on his brow! We continued to chat, and when I learned he had never been to a fashion show, I invited him and his wife to mine the following September.

As fashion week approached, Sergey called me with an intriguing offer: "What if you introduced Google Glass on the runway?" I almost fell out of my chair. I would be launching Google Glass? I thought it was a fantastic idea. My design and PR teams did not. "It's going to distract from the clothes and ruin the show," they claimed. "Wait a minute," I interrupted. "What is the main purpose of a show? To get beautiful photographs, right? Not only will we introduce this incredible technology that has never been seen, but we will be making a film that has never been made before: from the point of view of the models on the catwalk!" I also saw it as my secret weapon to turn around a show I was not feeling great about.

Indeed, it became a historic moment, especially when I grabbed Sergey from the audience to take the victory walk. The show was on every evening news broadcast around the world and the film, *DVF [through Google Glass]* was seen by millions on YouTube. Google Glass saved the day.

Yvan and I parted soon afterward. What we had to do to get the brand back on track would compromise his creativity. Joel insisted that I step back in to be the creative director and lead the designs back to our DNA. "What better person to do DVF than DVF?" he argued. Easier said than done. It took me more than a year to regain my confidence, find clarity, and slowly and painfully bring us back on brand.

One morning, my friend François-Marie Banier called me from Paris. He must have felt that I was insecure, and said something enlightening to me: "*assume-toi*," a French expression that means own yourself. What he was telling me was "Trust your own talent, learn to respect it." He was absolutely right. Though I always tell others "Dare to be you," I wasn't applying it to myself. "Make me a drawing of it, to remind me," I told him, laughing. That drawing now hangs on the wall next to my desk.

As I got much more involved in the creative process, Joel reorganized the company into divisions, with a unified team between design, merchandising, and sales, and a clear, nine-month time frame for design development. He hired a president of retail, a division head of accessories, a chief operating officer, our first chief marketing officer, and several others.

Joel also took it upon himself to ask each executive to define the DVF woman in one sentence. To his mounting frustration, he got a different answer each time, so he organized a focus session with Trey.

The goal of the daylong brainstorm was to come up with three words that exemplified DVF. Three words to identify our brand, our customer, and our designs. I was skeptical. We formed different groups and broke down words and sentences. Joel locked us in a room with coffee and pizzas so we wouldn't lose our momentum. By the end of the day I was surprised to see how many of the different groups came up with the same words: effortless, sexy, and on-the-go. Everyone applauded.

When the fog lifts, all of a sudden you see the light and everything becomes easier. Those three words brought us clarity. If it isn't effortless, if it isn't sexy, if you cannot put it in a little suitcase, it's not DVF. By the next day Joel was inundated with suggestions about what we had to do next, how to relate this definition to every facet of the business. Design and merchandising went back to edit the next collection with a new lens.

Joel's son found some old Ron Galella paparazzi pictures of me in a blur of motion, and Joel declared that's what DVF's image should be: on-the-go and caught in the moment. "She's glamorous, she's crossing the street, her hair is flying and she looks like somebody you want to be," he said. We needed to find the right model who was sophisticated and had confident body language—a girl who resembled, in a sense, the woman that I'd always wanted to become.

I turned to Edward Enninful, the talented fashion director of *W* magazine, whom I love and respect so much. "Who do you think should be in my ads?" I emailed him. Within the hour he responded with photographs of me as a young woman he'd pulled from the Internet alongside pictures of Daria Werbowy.

And there she was: a thirty-one-year-old Canadian woman of Ukrainian descent, extraordinarily beautiful and interesting-looking with long legs and wide-set blue eyes. Although she appears on the covers of *Vogue* worldwide, Daria is not your average supermodel. You never see her at parties, she is a world traveler, a hiker. She is the epitome of cool.

Daria's first DVF campaign was evocative and gritty. Night in New York. A beautiful young woman alone, confident, knowing where she is going, glancing behind her. "The images channel seventies-era paparazzi shots," wrote *Women's Wear Daily*, "with a spotlight on DVF's iconic wrap dresses." I knew we were on the right track.

As insurance that we didn't stray again, Paula brought in Stefani Greenfield, the friend who had originally brought Paula to me. Stefani, who sold Scoop in 2008 and now has her own consulting firm, understands the brand perfectly. Furthermore, she personally has a huge collection of DVF products and I was delighted to have her by our side.

Through all these transitions, many drawing from the strengths of the past and streamlining them for the future, was the unbelievable reality that in 2014 the wrap dress was turning forty! Joel called a meeting to discuss ideas for its birthday. Focusing on the wrap dress seemed a déjà vu for Paula and me. We needed to be convinced, but the young girls in marketing, and Stefani, were excited. Ideas were brought to the table: an exhibition, some collaborations.

As I started to think more and more about the dress I had created decades ago, and that was still selling, I realized I had always taken it for granted. Sometimes I even resented it when people talked about it as if it were the only thing I had ever done. Slowly but surely I began to look at it with fresh eyes and appreciated not only what it had done for me but also the value of the design itself. Effortless, sexy, and on-the-go, that little dress was very much the spirit of the brand! I decided to design a new one as an anniversary present to the original that had paid all my bills and had become part of fashion history.

In our line, we had a fit-and-flare dress that was very popular with young women, the Jeannie, named for our superstar head of production. Sleeveless, fitted stretch knit top, a flared skirt. It is simple and comfortable, sexy and effortless, easy to dress up or dress down. It quickly became a bestseller. When Victoria Beckham came to lunch at my office one day, she noticed it on a girl in the elevator and, after touching the easy stretch fabric, ordered one for herself on the spot.

If that flared skirt is so popular, I thought, I should turn it into a wrap dress. So I went to the sample room and called in Emily, the talented young woman I had discovered at the Savannah College of Art and Design when I spoke there at graduation years ago. I had noticed the simple but clever long jersey dress she had designed to wear for the occasion and offered her an internship. Emily has been working with us ever since. I told her that we would do this new wrap dress together. I explained that the top had to feel like a ballerina cover-up: tight jersey to flatter the bust and pinch the waist. For the circle skirt we chose a woven fabric that holds its shape well, but is still light.

We set to work building it and we fit it until it was perfect, just as I'd done with the first wrap dress in the factory outside Florence forty years before. I wanted to name the dress Emily, but along the way it became Amelia instead. We reissued the original snake print, the one that had danced down the runway at the Cotillion Room of the Pierre Hotel, and used it to make the new Amelia wrap. At first, our sales department did not even notice the dress; it had come so late that they barely showed it to buyers. In spite of my insecurity at the time, I forced our retail stores to buy it. I was right, Amelia was a hit, got a full page in *Vogue,* and became a bestseller! Reliving the magic with the birth of a new wrap, I became convinced. We would celebrate her fortieth birthday with pride. I was totally on board and excited when we all met again.

It was more or less at that time, as I started to regain my confidence and excitement, that Paula came to me and hinted that she wanted to leave. She was tired and felt it was time for her to look for a new horizon and new challenges. At first I refused to believe it; I always thought we were joined at the hip, that she was my partner in crime. We had built the new company. We were the Comeback Kids. "I can't imagine you not being here," I said. As she continued to discuss our separation with Joel, I slowly started to accept that she would leave.

Plans for the anniversary were accelerating. We decided to mount an exhibition and this time it would really earn its name: Journey of a Dress. It would be only about wraps: vintage wraps from the archives, current wraps, and we would create some anniversary wraps. A collaboration with Andy Warhol immediately came to my mind. What would be more DVF, more seventies yet modern than a Warhol wrap dress?

The first big decision was where to mount the exhibition. Los Angeles was my choice ... not only is it a city I love and where both my children live, but it has the right mixture of edginess, style, and pop culture. I love the light in LA, that very light that attracted the movie industry in the 1930s, a light that reinforces colors and boldness.

I made an appointment to see Michael Govan, the dynamic leader of the Los Angeles County Museum of Art (LACMA) and husband of the equally dynamic Katharine Ross, the superstar of fashion communications—art, fashion, and culture in one couple. In the museum parking lot, I got cold feet. "What am I going to tell him? Let's cancel," I told Grace Cha, my trusted VP of global communications. "We're already here," she said, incredulous. "Let's go in." And so in we went.

Of course as soon I began talking to Michael my adrenaline started racing. I relived the success of the exhibition in Beijing and how I had commissioned Chinese artists for it. I could feel his excitement and, with nothing to lose, I asked him, "How can I make this happen within your world? Do you know of any space near LACMA that I could use?" "Maybe," he said smiling.

The old May Company department store building sits on the LACMA campus and they had been using it for storage. They had begun clearing it out as it was going to be rebuilt by mega architect Renzo Piano into the spectacular Academy Museum of Motion Pictures. "You should meet with the Academy people and ask them," Michael suggested. "The timing may very well work for you."

An old famous department store on the LACMA campus that will become the museum of the film Academy? Was I dreaming? It sounded perfect!

When I entered the movie poster–lined hallways of the Academy to meet Dawn Hudson, the CEO, and Bill Kramer, director of development for their future museum, I was determined to seduce them. I guess Dawn felt the same way. She was wearing a DVF top, which I considered a good omen. She suggested we see the space, and if we liked it, she would ask the board.

The big, gloomy storage building was divided into endless large rooms packed with crates of art. It wasn't a pretty sight but I knew my friend interior designer Bill Katz could turn this gloom into glamour. It was full speed ahead.

What I did not know is that the Warhol Museum in Pittsburgh, where I'd never been, was also planning an anniversary, its twentieth. When Eric Shiner, the director, called to invite me to participate, he mentioned that there were lots of photos of me in their archives, and it tickled my curiosity. The next night, I ran into my good friend Bob Colacello, who had been *Interview* magazine's editor in the Warhol years, and as close to Andy as anyone could be. Stars were lining up and I decided to organize a field trip to Pittsburgh with Bill Katz, his assistant Kol, and Bob so that ideas for the exhibition would start to gel. But before that, I wanted Bob to take me on a day trip to Brooklyn to visit some young local artists. He planned the day guided by Vito Schnabel, Julian Schnabel's son, who is a successful independent art curator. As we visited the Bruce High Quality Foundation and Rashid Johnson's studio, I explained Journey of a Dress, and how I wanted to incorporate young artists in it. I invited Vito to come to Pittsburgh, too.

We took off early in the morning to fit in a visit to Fallingwater, Frank Lloyd Wright's beautiful nature-intensive house that I had always wanted to see, have a picnic on the way, and end up at Andy Warhol's museum in downtown Pittsburgh. We toured the museum, marveled at the paintings, watched the movies, and ended up in the private archive rooms where Eric had pulled out all of the photos

Andy had taken of me over the years. Bob and I felt as if we were back at Warhol's Factory.

For a few weeks I continued to visit artists' studios with Vito. I commissioned Dustin Yellin to make me a sculpture the minute I entered his studio in Red Hook, Brooklyn. He had never heard of the wrap dress, so I gave him a wrap for his girlfriend. Apparently he wore it around his studio instead, seeking inspiration from my early motto: "Feel like a woman, wear a dress!" I guess it worked, because he created a stunning 3D collage of the wrap frozen midmotion without a body inside. The "dress" is made up of hundreds, probably thousands of tiny, scanned black-and-white paper images of prints and newspaper articles cut into the shape of my first link print and laminated on multiple layers of glass inside a glass case. The dress floated in what looked like an aquarium to me and was the perfect blend of art and the wrap. Finding similar concepts with other artists, however, was getting very cerebral and confusing.

"Don't make it too complicated," Bill scolded me. "This exhibition has to be about the dress and about you. The art should only be from artists who have known you, painted you, worked with you . . . it is your journey and the journey of the dress. That is what this show has to be about. Use your bold prints, honor them, paste them on the walls, on the floors! Don't be shy!" Bill is the most visually secure person I know . . . no wonder Jasper Johns, Anselm Kiefer, and Francesco Clemente don't hang a painting without his advice. I was convinced. I kissed him.

Next, we met with Stefan Beckman, who designs the magnificent sets for Marc Jacobs's runway shows, and that was when the exhibit started to find its shape: we would have a time line, an art room, and one big room with an army of mannequins. I had always said I wanted an army of wraps, like the terra-cotta army of warriors I had seen in

Xi'an, China; a huge army of mannequins wearing the wraps. We'd started that idea with a group of thirty-six in Beijing, but I wanted many more for LA. I took Stefan to the mannequin manufacturer Ralph Pucci, whose in-house sculptor proceeded to design a mannequin by studying old photos of my face. He brought them to life with high cheekbones and, at my request, strong noses. I also wanted the mannequins to have a powerful pose, and so they did, inspired by the contrapposto of Michelangelo's *David*. I went many times to check on how those mannequins were evolving, and when I was satisfied that they looked strong and fearless, I ordered 225 of them.

Stefan designed the display of the mannequins, which would be divided into five diamond-shaped pyramids: a large one in the middle and four smaller ones around it. On the floor around the diamonds would be wide stripes of six "hero" prints chosen from the archives that we now call the six sisters: the nature-inspired Twigs, the geometric Cubes and Chain Link, the Leopard and Python, and the graphic print of my Signature. They would be greatly enlarged, printed on vinyl, and run across the floor and up the walls, making the whole thing look like a flag. I was thrilled. I had always wanted us to have a flag!

Now that Bill and Kol were designing the rooms, Stefan the sets, and Pucci the mannequins, Franca Dantes, our valuable archivist, was pulling images for the time line: Diana Vreeland's 1970 letter of encouragement, early advertisements, and memorable photos of women in wraps—everyone from Madonna to Ingrid Betancourt to Michelle Obama to Cybill Shepherd in *Taxi Driver*, Penélope Cruz in *Broken Embraces*, and Amy Adams in *American Hustle*. For the art room we would send all the works by Warhol, Francesco Clemente, Anh Duong, a new work by Barbara Kruger, photos by Helmut Newton, Chuck Close, Mario Testino, Horst, Annie Leibovitz, and the contemporary works we had commissioned for China. Luisella, once my assistant and now our VP of global events and philanthropy, was working on the logistics with Jeffrey Hatfield, our production person who had done Moscow, São Paulo, and Beijing. We were almost set except I did not have the most important link: Who was going to curate the dresses? Who was going to look at our huge archives, make sense of it all, and put it in a clear presentation? I certainly could not do that nor could anyone at DVF. For us they were just a bunch of old dresses!

Serendipity presented the answer. In June 2013 I went to England with my granddaughter Antonia to her boarding school orientation day, and to celebrate the eightieth birthday of Bob Miller, the founder of Duty Free shops and my cograndparent of Talita and Tassilo. When I go to London, I often take the opportunity to meet designers, to evaluate the pool of talent available. One of them was Michael Herz, creative director for Bally Switzerland.

We had met many years before when he was still a student and had a conversation sitting outside the Victoria & Albert Museum. This time, we had tea and a pleasant chat at Claridge's. He confessed that I always appeared on his inspiration boards. I liked his humorous take on things and I loved his description of women. There was poetry in everything he said and I was intrigued. He told me he was finishing his contract and would be taking time off. "It would be fun to do a project together," I said, having no idea what the project could be.

The moment I landed back in New York, I called Michael. "I may have a project for you," I said, and I invited him to Cloudwalk for the following weekend. Maybe he could curate the exhibition.

When Michael walked into my archive room and started putting the dresses on himself, I smiled. I left him to work alone for two days, to absorb it all. His first selection was very interesting. He had pulled out dresses I hadn't seen in years. He had spent hours in the old press books, taking photos, making notes, and sketching. By the end of his stay, I knew he should curate the show. "You have three months, three months to divide the dresses into groups and make sense of it all. I want you to mix them, old ones, new ones, and show the timelessness and the relevancy of the dress. You are allowed to reissue old prints, play with scales, and design new dresses . . . but it has to be seamless and effortless." He worked for one month alone and then we took two long days to go over it together.

Michael showed me the groups he wanted to do. The huge central diamond would be black-and-white dresses. "Black-and-white is perfect, but only if you mix it with colors. Black-and-white mixed with bright color, that is very DVF," I insisted. The other groups' themes were Nature, Animal, Geometric, and Pop. We rearranged them many times and he showed me sketches and the fabrics he wanted to reissue. I loved his choices. He disappeared into the sample rooms and factories for weeks. I let him do his thing, thinking I always had time to edit later.

The opening was planned for Friday, January 10, 2014, two days before the Golden Globe Awards. Eran Cohen, our new, much-needed CMO, and his team were in full planning now: construction, marketing, PR, and, last but not least, party planning.

When I went to check on the progress in early December, we met with the party planner but I was frustrated. I refused to have the party in a tent outside. I wanted the party to be inside, yet not in the exhibition. That is when I spotted an extra space adjacent to the large mannequin room and decided to convert its thirty-seven-hundred-square feet into my own Studio 54 with banquettes, mirrored columns, and disco balls!

Everything was in motion, no turning back.

Jeff and his team had started the construction after Thanksgiving and were going nonstop through all the holidays. The art was on the road, the new dresses were being made, and the old ones assembled. Franca was getting rights for the photos for the time line. Luisella, the grand conductor of it all, wanted to be on site. So she took Lensa, her adorable four-year-old daughter who is also my goddaughter, to LA to spend the holidays.

During the holiday while with my family on the boat, I kept pestering Jeffrey to send me photos. I was terrified that plastering the prints on the walls and floors would be too much. I flew back on January 2 and went straight from the plane to the museum. The space was magnificent and there was excitement in the air. The prints were on the floors and, although very bold, it looked almost neutral. I loved it.

We were still debating about the time-line gallery: pink walls? white walls? white floor? chain link floor? When Bill arrived the next day, everything crystallized. There was no more doubt. Pink walls. Chain link floor. Black and white and pink, the core colors of DVF. He started to hang the art, placed the Dustin Yellin in the middle of the time-line gallery and the original picture I had signed on the white cube in the entrance hall under the quote: "Fashion is a mysterious energy, a visual moment—impossible to predict where it goes."

Franca was sorting out the photos Bill wanted posted in the gallery. Michael was in the side rooms with dozens of interns, dressing the army of mannequins. Looking at the gallery that was shaping up, I decided that I wanted "Feel like a woman, wear a dress!" in neon right above the entrance. Jeffrey made it happen. We needed benches. He made that happen, too. As I walked through the dressed mannequins, I was in awe. I changed almost nothing of Michael's curation—except for the very central dress, at the front of the first big pyramid. I had a revelation: "We need the original black-and-white leopard!" I remembered that on my last trip to Miami, at the opening of the new Coral Gables store, a woman had walked in wearing it. I had looked at the label and confirmed that it was an original: 1974. She was very proud. "Call Adis, the Miami manager, and see if she can track that lady down. See if she will agree to lend it." She did.

Everything was ready.

Friday, January 10, 2014

I woke up early. Barry was asleep next to me, calm and reassuring. There we were, in the same bedroom where I landed thirty-nine years before. So much had happened and nothing had changed.

Before getting up, I lay still, imagining the day. A press conference was scheduled for 9:00 a.m. followed by a series of one-to-one interviews in different languages that would take most of the day. I had lined up different outfits in order to not look the same in all the photos. For the night, I had chosen a long black gown called the Geisha Wrap, a glamorous dress with dramatic sleeves and an obi sash lined in chartreuse silk.

I got up and, as I ate a bowl of pomegranate seeds, saw my face in the mirror. My eyes were puffy. Not a good start. I put on a mask and got into the steam shower. As usual, I did my own hair and waited for Sarah, the makeup artist, to arrive, though the last thing I wanted was to put on makeup. Sarah's touch was light and slowly I started to feel better.

I put on my python jacquard pants, my camouflage leopard shirt, my leather jacket, and my booties, and kissed Barry goodbye. I took the clothes I had prepared and everything I would need to survive the press day and threw it all in the car.

Off I went in my little rental Mercedes. As I drove down Sunset Boulevard, turning on Fairfax, I checked myself in the mirror and winked. As I arrived at Wilshire, I saw the huge building with large banners of my face by Warhol all around it. "Dianette," I told myself in French, "Your whole life is in that box!" I smiled.

Walking into the long time-line gallery, my clothes over my arm, I felt like the Diane who used to love walking into Studio 54 alone, feeling like a pioneer in a saloon, confident, with the desire to conquer . . . a man's life in a woman's body.

I went into the back office where, in the chaos of the last-minute preparations, I changed into a little black-and-white dress, nude fishnet stockings, and high-heeled sandals . . . feel like a woman, wear a dress!

Inside my shoe, for good luck, I scotch-taped one of my father's gold coins, the ones he smuggled into Switzerland in 1942. For a moment, I closed my eyes and I felt thankful.

Thankful to God for having saved my mother,

To my mother for giving me life,

To my children for being who they are,

To Barry for always being there for me.

I was then ready for the day, ready to honor the little dress that started it all.

Everyone came to the party. Like a cast at the end of a movie, all the actors of my life showed up.

My modern family first: Barry; my children, Alexandre and Tatiana, with their significant others; Ali Kay; Russell Steinberg; Francesca Gregorini; Alexandra and her companion, Dax. My granddaughter Antonia was unfortunately at boarding school and Leon was too small to show up, but Tassilo was there with Talita and her friends, who represented the new generation of wrap girls in their DVF/Andy Warhol dresses. My brother, Philippe, his wife, Greta, and his daughters Sarah and Kelly flew in from Belgium; Martin Muller from San Francisco; Ginevra Elkann from Rome; Olivier Gelbsmann and Hamilton South from New York; Konstantine Kakanias and Nona Summers.

TV host extraordinaire Andy Cohen and model Coco Rocha welcomed all the guests on the red carpet, and we live-streamed their arrival. California governor Jerry Brown and his wife, Anne, followed by my fashion friends Anna Wintour, André Leon Talley, and Hamish Bowles. Then came my actor friends, Gwyneth Paltrow; Raquel Welch; Demi Moore; Rooney Mara; Robin Wright and her daughter, Shauna; Tobey Maguire and his designer wife, Jennifer Meyer; Julie Delpy; Ed Norton; Seth Meyers; Allison Williams; and the Hilton sisters. Hollywood aristocracy was represented by David Geffen, Bryan Lourd, Sandy Gallin, and many more. My American friends Anderson Cooper, restaurateur Bruce Bozzi, Amazon's Jeff Bezos and his wife; CFDA's Steven Kolb; Alyse Nelson from Vital Voices; Vito Schnabel; Dustin Yellin and Bob Colacello; Linda Bird Francke. Joel Horowitz led the DVF contingent with Stefani Greenfield and many DVF executives, as well as Ellen, my loyal assistant who came back to my side as my chief of staff. My first boss, Albert Koski, and his wife,

Danièle Thompson, flew in from Paris, as did Christian Louboutin, François-Marie Banier, Martin d'Orgeval, and Johnny Pigozzi.

The exhibit was a huge success and lasted for four months. Almost 100,000 visitors, tens of thousands of posts on social media, rave reviews from all over the world. Even the most critical fashion experts loved it and acknowledged the undeniable timelessness of the dress and its infinite versatility. It was no longer just about the past, but also about the future.

It had a great impact on the business and created a demand for the wraps for yet another generation. But for all the effects it had on others, the most surprising and exciting is the effect it had on me. Seeing the body of my work in that show made me so proud and, for the first time ever, I felt totally legitimate. It propelled me into what I call the new era, the next chapter of my company that will last after me.

Like my life, my work has been a wonderful adventure. It allowed me to become the woman I wanted to be as I helped other women to feel the same. I went into it looking for confidence and spread confidence along the way.

I don't know if I have reached wisdom, but hopefully my experiences, told with all the honesty and candor I could find in my heart and in my memory, will inspire others to take their lives in their hands, be their best friends, and go for it fearlessly.

About the Author

DIANE VON FURSTENBERG first entered the fashion world in 1972 with a suitcase full of jersey dresses. Two years later, she created the wrap dress, which came to symbolize power and independence for an entire generation of women. By 1976, she had sold more than a million of the dresses and was featured on the cover of *Newsweek*. After a hiatus from fashion, Diane relaunched the iconic dress that started it all in 1997, reestablishing her company as the global luxury lifestyle brand that it is today. DVF is now sold in over fifty-five countries. In 2005, Diane received the Lifetime Achievement Award from the Council of Fashion Designers of America (CFDA) for her impact on fashion, and one year later was elected the CFDA's president, an office she continues to hold. In 2012, Diane was named the most powerful woman in fashion by *Forbes* magazine.